MY Special BROTHER

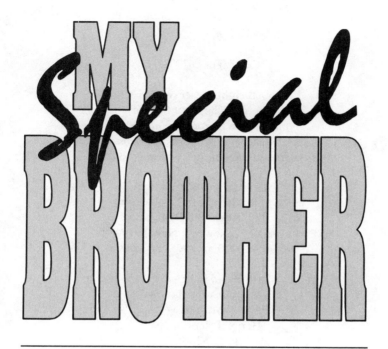

MY Special BROTHER

RENA SCHIFF

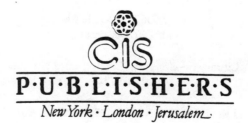

CIS
P·U·B·L·I·S·H·E·R·S
New York · London · Jerusalem

Published and distributed
in the U.S., Canada and overseas by
C.I.S. Publishers and Distributors
180 Park Avenue, Lakewood, New Jersey 08701
(908) 905-3000 Fax: (908) 367-6666

Distributed in Israel by
C.I.S. International (Israel)
Rechov Mishkalov 18
Har Nof, Jerusalem
Tel: 02-538-935

Distributed in the U.K. and Europe by
C.I.S. International (U.K.)
89 Craven Park Road
London N15 6AH, England
Tel: 01-809-3723

Book and cover design: Deenee Cohen
Typography: Chaya Bleier

ISBN 1-56062-102-8 hard cover
1-56062-101-X soft cover

Library of Congress Catalog Card Number
91-61774

PRINTED IN THE UNITED STATES OF AMERICA

This book is dedicated to
the parents of "Leibish"

Introduction

▼

There has been a single most important motivation behind this venture, and that was to bring the potential reader face to face with a child afflicted with Down Syndrome and with the people around him. If this book helps even one person smile to such a child, or any other unfortunate human being; if by reading this story he or she takes notice of disabled people, when otherwise this same person would have instinctively ignored them, this book will have been well worth it.

The story as well as the characters are all real, based on a true life story. For the purposes of writing this book, I have assumed the identinty of one of the daughters of the family, and I have projected my thoughts and feelings into the situation. Otherwise, I have remained as faithful as possible to the actual story as it occured. Some minor incidents and most of the names, except for the names of the staff at HASC, have been altered to protect the anonymity of the family involved.

First and foremost, I would like to thank the parents of "Leibish" without whom this book would have been impossible. May you have *nachas* from him and all your other children, grandchildren and great-grandchildren, *ad meah v'esrim shanah.*

Thank you, my dear husband, for your constant support and encouragement throughout this project.

Thank you, my dear parents for instilling in me the values and ethics that have enabled me to empathize so deeply with a child such as Leibish.

A special note of appreciation to the staff at HASC and STEP BY STEP.

Special thanks to Rabbi Reinman and Raizy Kaufman at CIS Publishers.

Rena Schiff

Table of Contents

▼

Great News

▼

April 20, 1964

Mommy told us the exciting news. She is going to have a baby in just a few short weeks! I decided this was the perfect time to start a diary. My English teacher claims I am very good at "creative writing" and always urges me to make use of my talent. I guess writing a diary is good practice. I wonder if I'll ever let anyone see it, or if with time, I will lose my enthusiasm. I hope not. It would be wonderful to look back many years from now and read all about myself and my family. Who knows? Maybe my children will even read it. Perhaps it will serve like a miniature history book for my family. I am really getting carried away with my dreams. But aren't dreams important in life? Tatty always talks about how important it is to dream. He says, "Dreams are the energy fueling our hopes and deeds. They help us strive for better things."

We are elated with the unexpected news. It's been seven years since Lezerl was born, and we have almost forgotten what it feels like to have a baby in the house. I am already eleven years old, and I feel I will be a great help—Mommy will just have to smile and coo at the baby, and the rest I could handle quite easily.

We are, *baruch Hashem*, a happy family. True, my parents are busy all week. Tatty holds down two jobs. During the day he is a *mashgiach* at a large restaurant, and on evenings and weekends, he caters at small affairs. When things get real busy in the catering business, we all help out.

Mommy works at a dress shop a few blocks away. Mommy hates wasting time. Even when not at work, she always finds something to do. She cooks, bakes, sews everything we wear and runs the house very efficiently. Although we are not rich, we never feel deprived; on the contrary, we feel very fortunate.

So when *Shabbos* arrives, it is a special treat. Everyone is home from work and school. The *Shabbos tisch* is a delight for everyone, as we catch up on missed conversations. The dining room fills with the lovely *zemiros* of my father with his sweet voice, accompanied by my two brothers. Mommy always has a wonderful story, and at bedtime she can always come up with a new little melody from "*di alte heim.*"

Thus when the announcement came today, we felt it was too good to be true. Preparations are under way. Not in the physical sense, of course, since our *minhag* dictates that nothing be prepared in advance. Rather, we are planning who'll be first to hold the baby, who will get to walk the baby, who will get to give the bottle to the baby. The word baby is on everyone's mind.

Our parents look on in amusement. "How lucky these kids are," they think. "They have none of the worries we carry around." Not that they worry about the financial aspect, or how they would handle another child. That is not the Jewish way.

Everyone knows that each child brings its own *mazel*. However, my parents, as any other parents, hope that it will be a healthy child that will grow up and give them much *nachas*.

Friday, July 3, 1964

This morning, we awoke to the shrill sound of the ringing telephone. As much as we thought we were prepared for the upcoming event, the phone call came as a real surprise. Etty, my "big sister," picked up the phone, and after a moment, we heard her scream, "It's a boy!" We all started jumping about and chanting excitedly "*Mazel tov!* It's a boy! It's a boy! Now we are even; three girls and three boys!"

Only Etty did not seem to share our excitement. There was something troubling in her eyes. I grew frightened. Was there something wrong with Mommy, Heaven forbid? That was too horrible to even imagine, and so I pushed that thought quickly out of my mind.

Was the baby . . .? No, no. It couldn't be. The baby was just fine. It had to be. Mommy and Tatty have suffered enough already. In those fleeting moments, as I stood there transfixed, I reflected on my parents' past.

Sara, my mother, grew up in a small town in Hungary. Her parents worked hard to support their large family. Her mother, who loved her children dearly, had no time nor strength to care for the little ones. They were left to fend for themselves.

Little Sara's childhood was rudely torn from her at a very

young age. She never knew what it meant to be a carefree little girl. There was work, work, and then some. In those days, a maid was not a luxury, it was a necessity. There were no vacuum cleaners, no washing machines, no permanent press fabrics. Everything had to be hand washed and ironed. But in my mother's home, there was no money for servants, and she would perfom tasks normally given to the maid. At an age when her friends were learning how to catch a ball and jump rope, Mommy was learning the basics of housework and the rudiments of *matzah*-baking. At the young age of eight, she began to work in her parents' *matzah* bakery. Right from when she returned from school, until late at night, Sara could be found working along with the hired workers. She had no time to study and no time to play with her friends.

Despite all the hardship and poverty, Mommy grew up a confident teenager with the whole world before her. She would allow nothing to stand in her way to happiness and fulfillment.

But her road to happiness was being blocked by something larger than life, more evil and more malevolent than anything the world had ever encountered. Hitler was blocking the road to happiness, the road to life itself, not only for Sara but for millions like her.

"Adversity breeds character," goes the saying, and indeed, the years of hardship and hard work came to her aid.

Sara, along with the other townspeople, was herded onto a truck headed to an unknown place from which everyone knew there would be little chance of returning. She looked hither and thither, and when she was certain no one was looking, she mustered all her courage and jumped off the truck! She landed on the soft ground, and losing no time, she took off like a bird, running so fast she felt as if she had grown wings.

Somehow, she obtained false papers, and with incredible determination, surprising even herself, she came through the horrors of the war, unscathed and whole.

There was one spark lighting her way through those terrible years. Chaim Weinfeld, her brother's long time *chavrusa*, had also obtained false papers and was hiding "underground," posing as a gentile. He used his position as a "free, roaming Hungarian gentile" to save countless Jews. He got hold of a large stack of Swiss papers replete with the Swiss insignia and distributed them to whichever Jew came his way. All they had to do was fill in a certain code, and they were on their way to safety. Many Jews owe thanks for their lives to the heroic young man who is my father. May this be in his *zchus* forever.

My parents would meet at the home of a Catholic couple who were of the small minority of gentiles sympathetic to the hapless Jews. There they would encourage each other to keep strong and never lose hope. Rumors had it that Hitler was being beaten and that the end was near. They must be patient and wait.

The waiting seemed endless, but come it did. Chaim and Sara were now orphans, their parents having been murdered along with their younger siblings. They were on their own, facing an uncertain future. There was no question what their next step would be. They had grown to respect each other over the years they had suffered together, keeping the secret of each other's Jewishness, never divulging it to anyone, not even other Jews. They always stayed Jews in their hearts, even while parading around as a couple of gentiles.

They had met through Torah when Chaim would visit my mother's home to study with her brother, chanting the sweet *Gemara nigun* together. They would meet again, under the *chupah*, to build a house filled with Torah and *Yiddishkeit*.

The years flew by. Chaim and Sara had five beautiful children. They moved to America and settled in Boro Park. They worked hard and earned an honest living. They were able to save up for a down payment on a comfortable home with a backyard and a front lawn. It was a dream come true, and certainly a triumph for a couple who had started all the way from the bottom.

I shook myself, as if to bring my mind back to the present. Could this be true? Could it be that things were not as happy as they should be? No, of course not. Mommy had a new baby, and we should be celebrating. We should be running to school to tell our friends. Our eyes should be shining, our hearts singing. We have a new baby, something we have long wished for, and we must enjoy every minute of it. I must tell Etty to take that glum look off her face. It does not suit the occasion.

Sunday, July 5, 1964

It's late, and I should really be in bed. I'm exhausted! But first I must continue writing about all that happened on Friday. I must get it off my chest, or I will burst. Usually, when something bothers me, I can always pour my heart out to Gitty. I talk to Gitty so much on the phone that when Tatty picks up the phone and hears Gitty's voice he calls, "Rochelle, it's Gitty Telephone!" (That is my father's nickname for her).

Somehow, these latest events are different. How I hope they will not change everything. I pray that my parents will be able to bear it without too much change to their personalities. My sister Raizy and I have made a pact. We will help as much as possible and lighten our dear parents' heavy load.

Well, let's get on with it. When Etty sensed something was wrong, that the news was turning out not quite as anticipated she asked, "Tatty, what's wrong? Please tell me."

"Well," Tatty answered evasively, "the doctors think there is something wrong with his neck. It is unusually thick."

"What does that mean?" Etty was alarmed at the turn of events.

"We are waiting for a conclusive report. The doctors are putting the baby through some tests."

When Tatty came home from the hospital to get the house ready for *Shabbos* and prepare for the *shalom zachar*, he went about everything in a daze. This was not our usual father who always loved a good joke and did everything cheerfully. It saddened us all, and everyone was unusually tense. This was not nearly as exciting as we had envisioned. No one could muster up the courage to ask what was so terrible about a thick neck.

The truth was, as it turned out later, that Tatty did know the meaning of "a thick neck." There was much more to it . . .

Despite everything, the *shalom zachar* in *shul* was a great success. There was lots of food and plenty of bottles of beer, which Tatty had placed earlier in the day into our bathtub filled with great chunks of ice. I must say my parents are very popular. One would think that in July, when many people are up in the mountains, there would hardly be a *minyan*. (This is the only time that I remember being in the city during the summer, the reason, of course, being the baby.) We were pleasantly surprised at the large turnout. At one point, even Tatty, busy greeting and serving his friends and relatives, looked so happy that I would like to think that for the moment he forgot the anxiety that had been with him all that day.

We came home from the *shalom zachar* late at night. The candles had long since burned out, and we were exhausted. We were all ready to fall into bed and contemplated how we would even manage to get into our pajamas without falling asleep.

Tatty had other plans, however. He instructed Lezer to go to sleep, and for once Lezer did not protest, as he usually did. He did not even claim that the clock was too fast, that it was really much earlier and that he was not tired! Tatty gathered the rest of us around the kitchen table, where the *Shabbos* light was still on, and began to speak.

"I know, *kinderlach*, that you are tired. The truth is that I am tired, too. Besides having been up all last night with Mommy, I had a rough day today. I'm sure you are looking forward to a good night's sleep just like I am. Funny, just when you do want to go to sleep I don't let you. I guess tonight is *venahapochu*. But isn't *Purim* still a long way off?"

We appreciated Tatty's attempt to add some humor to what was turning out quite the opposite. The mood was somber and strained, so we managed a little chuckle. It did little, however, to relieve the tension.

Tatty went on more seriously. "Allow me to have just a few words with you, and then we can all go and catch up on some much needed sleep. In my opinion, it is best not to hide things that concern all of us, the sooner we face the facts, the better we will cope. Lezer is still quite young, so I think there is no rush in burdening him with information he might not even fully understand and which might cause him needless concern. The rest of you are older, and being bright and intelligent, I am certain you will listen carefully to what I have to tell you and utilize the information properly."

It was so quiet in the room, you could hear the curtains rustling in the gentle summer night's breeze. We did not take our eyes off Tatty for a second. He went on, tears welling up in his dark green eyes.

"The doctors saw immediately that there was something wrong with the baby. First they said that he had a thick neck. Actually, his neck appears to be short and broad because of the extra skin and tissue at the base of the neck area. After they put him through a battery of physical and mental tests, much more elaborate than the standard tests they give every newborn, they confirmed that he is a mongoloid."

The word mongoloid struck at us with an unimaginable fierceness. It was an unspoken word that applied to *other* children, of *other* families. Our family was perfect. We were normal, healthy children. We all had many friends, both our parents and us, who always liked visiting our cheerful house. A mongoloid was someone living far away who looked funny, who hardly spoke, who was miles behind other children in everything, shunned by everyone around him. How could such a child now be part of us? Worse yet, how can we accept it without feeling the same way we felt when on rare occasions we would glimpse such a child and think, "How does this kid's mother take it? Aren't the siblings embarrassed of him?" This was all a bad dream. We should indeed go to sleep. Our imaginations were acting up badly tonight. However, sleep was furthest from our minds. We sat with our mouths open and hearts beating so loudly that we could hear every beat distinctly.

Tatty swallowed hard. It was clear he was having a hard time of it. He forced himself to continue, taking a deep breath.

"The doctor who delivered the baby saw our distress and

came over to us and said very gently, 'You have two choices. Put him in a home and forget him, or take him home and love him.' To me, there are no choices. When Mommy comes home, she will bring him. We will all share in this big task. We will do just as the doctor said. We will *love* him.

"There was one image that kept coming to my mind, dear children, when I discovered our baby's infirmity, and I could not shake it. Yossele."

"Who was Yossele, and what has he to do with our new baby?" we asked, curious.

Tatty closed his eyes, as if to bring back the past.

"The Golds lived behind the *shul* in the town of Helserd. Mendel Gold was the *shamess* in the *shul*. He was well liked, gentle and kind. The Golds had a child who was, *lo aleinu*, retarded. No one knew exactly what was wrong with him; they only knew that he was '*meshuga*.' Had Yossele been born fifty years later, he would have been diagnosed by professionals as 'mongoloid.' (His prominent facial characteristics were marked by the same small slanted eyes as the Mongols who invaded what is today Russia, thus the name 'mongolism.') With proper care and stimulation, his situation would have been entirely different. He most probably would have mastered at least some words, could have been trained, albeit later than normal children, and could have even helped his parents with some menial jobs around the house.

"However, it was Yossele's misfortune to have been born in a darker time. Yossele was treated worse than a dog. When he was small, he was fed some mush and then put in a room with a dirt floor, with no toys or any other articles, so that he shouldn't hurt anything or anyone. He spent the entire day there. Often, he would eat the dirt off the floor. He was not trained, and when he got dirty, he would roll in his own dirt. In the summer, he was allowed to be in a large pen, originally a chicken coop. There he would sit and sway to and fro all day . Every so often, he would venture out through the small trap door on his hands and knees, but he was quickly caught and put back in the pen.

"At age eight, he finally learned to walk, with an irregular, unsteady gait. His speech was limited to some unintelligible grunts, which no one bothered to try to understand. He was never dressed in anything but tattered pajamas, day and night, winter and summer, weekdays or holidays. When his walking was steadier, his ventures out of the pen and house became more frequent and farther from the house. When on several occasions he disappeared for long periods of time, the Golds believed there was only one solution—to place him in shackles! With the heavy iron chains attached to his ankles, Yossele could make only short, jerky steps."

Here we all gasped. We were sickened by this narrative and wondered why Tatty had to tell it in such detail. Tatty continued.

"One would think that the neighbors would protest this inhumane treatment. Interestingly enough, no one protested. Not that everyone in Helserd was cruel and unfeeling. The families in the *shtetl* were very close-knit, and the parents were devoted and caring to their children. So why this callousness? The sad fact was, that for children born '*meshuga*' (the terms mentally retarded, learning disabled, etc. were still unheard of, at least by the common folks), there was no hope. They would never amount to anything. They had to be guarded, like dangerous wild animals, to prevent them from harming themselves or others and were shunned by society. Without the proper guidance, these children did usually grow up resembling animals more closely than human beings.

"You see, children," Tatty concluded. "There is no limit to the destruction ignorance can foster. We will all pool our resources and try to help our little newcomer develop into a little *mentchele*. We will never call him, nor even think of him, *chas veshalom*, as '*meshuga*.' We will come to think of him as one of us, which he is, and accept his differences with love and understanding."

Tuesday, July 7, 1964

Today I ran to the library and did thorough research on mongolism. I want to write down briefly what I read, so that it will help me better understand our new brother's behavior, especially in the first crucial years. I never had any close personal encounters with such children, although I have read that it is not such a rare condition. In fact, it affects about one to two of every one hundred babies born.

Once one learns how the body and its many components operate one can fully appreciate what a masterpiece Hashem has created. Just like bricks make up a building, our bodies are made up of countless cells. There are millions of different cells that compose the different body parts. There are bone cells, marrow cells, skin cells, blood cells, etc. At the center of each cell, in the nucleus, is the master plan, from which messages are sent to the body to do certain things at certain times, like when a baby should sit up, where the eyes and other organs should be located and myriad other functions. The master plan is controlled by the chromosomes, which look like tiny threads.

Human beings have forty-six chromosomes in each cell, except for the red blood cells and the germ cells. They form twenty-three pairs of chromosomes. Sometimes, while the baby is developing inside the mother, as the cells divide and subdivide to form a healthy, normal baby, something goes awry and one of the cells does not divide fully, leaving one of the pairs of chromosomes "stuck together." This will form the extra chromosome, as the cell will have acquired a new, divided pair to replace the misaligned one.

This condition is called Down's Syndrome, named for Langdon Down who first identified it. Surprisingly, the name Down's Syndrome has only been in use for the last few years. Only five years ago, in 1959, it was discovered that the extra chromosome was responsible for this condition. Up until then, these children were referred to as mongols—as they still are by most people—because they look like the Oriental Mongols.

To tell the truth, I have photocopied the page in the encyclopedia that had this information and have written it down in a short, simple version. It is all very complicated and technical. I don't pretend to understand it all, but it has given me a vague picture of why our baby is the way he is. To think that an extra chromosome in the cells can do so much harm! What's more, it is as healthy as the other chromosomes. Since everything in the body is controlled by these chromosomes it is easy to comprehend why, when there is a deviation in their number, everything in the body will be affected.

As a woman gets older, her chances of giving birth to a child with Down's Syndrome will increase. Not that Mommy is so old. Interestingly enough, when it comes to giving birth, thirty-five is already considered older. Although there is always a chance that a woman at any age will have a baby with some form of handicap, statistically, the chances of something going wrong with the baby increase dramatically with age.

Now that I've read about the visual signs of these babies, I am certain Mommy knew right away that something was wrong. No wonder she is so depressed, she won't even speak to us on the phone! She must have seen the typical short broad hands, with their distinctive crease patterns—the palm of the hand will usually have only one crease instead of the usual two. Even more recognizable are their faces. I'm sure mongoloid children each have their individual looks, our baby being especially cute. Their parents' genes get passed along to them much the same as all babies, but there are certain characteristics that are typical. They have puffy eye lids; their eyes slope upwards at the outer corners; the face and features are small; the tongue is sometimes enlarged, with weak muscle tone, and tends to stick out; their mouths are unusually small, aggravating this condition and making feeding especially difficult. Nursing these babies is sometimes very difficult. When they are older, the enlarged tongue, coupled by at least some degree of retardation, results in many feeding problems. They have to be taught to take the food off the spoon and swallow it, a very difficult task for the very young mongoloid child.

Although not all babies with this condition have all the above-mentioned characteristics, I was devastated to learn that *all* these children are born mentally retarded. The words stung. I know, however, that the term is broad, that even amongst these children there are dramatic differences in their functioning levels, ranging from very low to high functioning. I determined that, with our efforts, we will minimize his infirmities dramatically and help him achieve his full potential. As if to confirm my thoughts, I was relieved to read that, if brought up in a normal family environment and given plenty of love and attention, they can grow up to be happy, active participants in family life because they are very responsive, loving and even-tempered.

I have always heard that mongoloid children did not live long. In 1929, their average life expectancy was only nine years! Only ten years ago, it was nineteen years. There is growing evidence that with proper care, medical and mental, they could live well into adulthood.

As I read on, I felt like I was riding a roller coaster. Just as I glimpsed at some hopeful facts, I was thrown into despair once again. It scared me to discover that these babies are especially prone to some diseases, particularly to respiratory and ear infections, due to a weak immune system. About a third have some form of congenital heart disease. Since no one mentioned, Heaven forbid, anything about our baby's heart, I am led to believe that, *baruch Hashem*, our baby is okay in that respect.

We must learn to appreciate the positive and cope optimistically with the negative aspects. As Mommy always says, "One must look up in hope, and never forget to look down—and see how much worse it could have been."

Friday, July 10, 1964

Yesterday, Mommy and the baby came home. We all had mixed feelings. We looked forward to having Mommy back home and were also excited and anxious to see our new baby. What would he look like? How would Mommy handle all this?

The only one who seems oblivious to all this is Lezer. He

does not seem to notice anything unusual and is perfectly happy. He acts like any other seven-year-old with a new baby in the house. The recent *shalom zachar* and the anticipation of the *vach nacht* and *bris*, are all very exciting to Lezer, especially all the *pekelech* he plans to give out at the *vach nacht* to all the little children who will come to say *shema*.

The *bris* should have been this morning, but the *mohel* says the baby is "yellow." I wonder if this has anything to do with his disorder. Even though I know that yellowness is a type of jaundice with which many children are born, I find myself blaming everything on "it."

When Mommy came home, we looked expectantly at her to see any signs of distress. We were relieved to see that she looked quite cheerful. As we spoke, I began to realize that she did not seem to believe there was anything wrong with the baby. Indeed, as we looked into the little crib where the baby lay peacefully asleep, we almost believed it, too. The thought that this was all a bad dream, that this baby was perfect, kept playing on our minds repeatedly. "Wishful thinking" took on lifesize meaning.

Later, when everyone else was asleep, I lay awake listening to my parents' gloomy discussion in the other room.

"Sara, I'm happy you're acting to our new baby just like you did to our other babies," Tatty was saying. "But I want you to realize he is different. Not that I want to upset you. You know I always mean well and want you to be happy. But the sooner you accept the truth, the easier it will be for you to adjust."

"No, no!" my mother almost shouted, pleadingly. "Look at him, so sweet and cuddly. It can't be true! Those heartless doctors, what do they really know? Oh, I admit he does look different from my other children, and his eyes are a little slanted.

But I'm sure, in time, his features will straighten out, and he will be just a regular boy. It can't be any other way. I can't bear it that *my child*, whom I carried for nine long difficult months and whom I love, is not normal, *chas veshalom*. I believe Hashem can do wonders. He will make sure our baby will turn out okay.

"The doctors act as if they are G-d. I will never forget the indifference of the resident doctor when he told us right after the birth, 'Just place him in a mental institution and forget you ever had him. Go home and enjoy the rest of the children. Why bother suffering? He'll never talk, may never be trained and, possibly, may never even walk. You can expect him to live no longer than fourteen years.' The doctor made the baby sound like an unwanted package. Can't he see that the baby is as human as anyone? I don't believe there is anything wrong with him, and it must all be a terrible mistake."

"But what about the doctors' diagnosis?" Tatty insisted. "They ran a whole battery of tests on him and confirmed their suspicion one hundred percent. We even had Dr. Metz, the nationally acclaimed pediatrician from Manhattan, come down to see the baby and he, too, confirmed their diagnosis."

But Mommy held fast to her belief. Obviously, she could not bring herself to face the truth.

Later, Tatty walked over to the crib where the infant lay peacefully asleep, and looked down lovingly at his newborn son. He spoke to the child, his voice full of love and concern.

"Listen carefully, little one. I love you just like I love my other children, maybe even more. I know you are different, but nevertheless, it does not change my feelings towards you. On the contrary, I feel a special responsibility to make life as easy and enjoyable as possible for you. It is not your fault that you were born this way. I will always keep that in mind."

Tatty sounded all choked up with emotion. I cried and cried for him and for Mommy and for all of us until I fell into a restless sleep.

A Full Time Job

Tuesday, January 12, 1965

Mothers like to tell you what a full-time job having a baby is. Well, if a baby is a full-time job, then a special baby is an overflowing full-time job, and then some. We are all so busy with the baby, far more than we had ever dreamed. How could I have been afraid that no one would let me help, that I would end up begging Mommy to let me feed it? There is so much to do, more than enough for everyone. Anyone in the family who is willing to help is welcome. Mommy has made it clear that she will not allow Leibish to hinder us in any way. Aside from certain chores we were always assigned, and that according to our ages we are obligated to perform, as in any normal household, everything is on a strictly voluntary basis. She will never let us forego our Bnos group on *Shabbos* or any school trips.

However, there is one thing she made very clear. She firmly believes that "charity begins at home." Countless times, my mother has taught us what *mitzvos* are all about. She did not

29

learn Ramban and Malbim, as we do today. There was no Bais
Yaakov, at least not in her parts. But sometimes, I think she has
it all straighter than we do. She tells us that, somehow, people
like the "glorious" *mitzvos*, the ones that are noble and prominent. No wonder we are told in *Pirkei Avos*, "Be careful with the
light *mitzvos* as you would be with the weighty." It is so much
more gratifying to save someone from drowning than to protect
a friend from needless shame. Who are we to judge which
mitzvah is more important, saving a life or saving face? There
is no minimum when it comes to doing a *chessed* with your
fellow man. Helping a sister who has little children and has a
hard time coping is just as important as doing *chessed* the "big
way," like going with a large group of girls to an old age home.
Mommy is always teaching this to us, as she feels the priorities
today are sometimes mixed up.

Picture this: Mrs. Klein asks Shaindy, her downstairs neighbor, to babysit for her. It is *Shabbos* morning, her regular
babysitter has not shown up, and she is in a bind. Her youngest
sister is having *sheva berachos*, and she has no other way to
leave her little ones. A look of supreme holiness descends on
Shaindy's face. Her neighbor literally begs her to come up. She
promises it will only be for an hour or two. But Shaindy
solemnly explains, "I'm sorry, Mrs. Klein, but I don't babysit on
Shabbos. It is against my principles." Perhaps this commands
great respect from her neighbor, but when the door closes and
Mrs. Klein finds herself inside her apartment once again, she
buries her head in her pillow and cries her heart out. She must
stay home when everyone else in the family is having a good
time at her youngest sibling's *sheva berachos*.

That same girl who does not babysit on *Shabbos*, goes off
after the *seudah* to visit a sick woman who is bedridden and

looks forward to the "nice girls" who come to see her every *Shabbos*. It is all very virtuous and kind of Shaindy; she is a true *baalas chessed*. Little does she realize, however, that by babysitting for her neighbor, she would have done, perhaps, an even greater kindness. Had she answered, "I will gladly do it, if you have no other way of joining your family's *simchah*. But being that it is *Shabbos*, I will do it for you as one neighbor to another, not as a job."

Our friends at school have signed up this year to go "patterning." These are special exercises performed with children who are severely handicapped and would lie as vegetables if not stimulated physically. This immobility may threaten their health and make them susceptible to pneumonia and muscle atrophy, *chas veshalom*. The girls are all proud to have joined the "*Bikur Cholim* Gang." Every lunch hour a different group of girls goes to a house with a sick child, *lo aleinu*, and proceeds with an exercise routine.

Raizy went last year, as she was already in high school. When she came home after the first time, she looked drawn and very pale. I asked her what had happened, and she told me she had gone patterning at a family by the name of Halberstam, and she got the part where she had to turn the boy's head from one side to another. There were four more girls, each taking one limb.

It went something like this. The left foot and left hand were flexed upwards, while the right foot and hand were simultaneously bent downwards. Aryele's head was turned to the side which was down. Much like the crawl stroke at swimming. This kept the whole body in motion, and it was thought that this would artificially stimulate the brain cells which would normally move these muscles naturally. Eventually, it was hoped that these cells would sort of "spring to life" and resume these movements on their own.

The problem was that Aryele, about the age of six or seven, kept drooling on Raizy's hands. His mouth muscles were apparently just as lax as the rest of the muscles in his wasted body. Raizy had tried to ignore it and kept a cheerful disposition. She was the only one who knew the type of Yiddish Aryele was spoken to, and though he was mentally disabled as well, he smiled his sweet innocent smile as she sang him some songs she had learned from our mother and made little jokes with him. His eyes were shining, as though expressing his appreciation for this entertainment. Raizy couldn't contain herself any longer. The tears were running down her cheeks. Her heart ached for this innocent little boy whose suffering was so great.

Just then Aryele's mother came into the room, and Raizy quickly wiped her tears so that she should not see her crying. Mrs. Halberstam had enough sorrow to deal with, and Raizy was there to lighten the burden, not aggravate it.

Now that we had a child in our family who needed special care and stimulation, Mommy explained that it made sense for us to perform our *bikur cholim mitzvos* right here in this very house. We had a built-in *mitzvah*, and we did not have to run far to find it.

Working with Leibish is very rewarding and I feel gratified to earn so many *mitzvos*. Had Mommy pushed us into it, I probably would have resented it and would have tried at every opportunity to get away from it. Mommy's attitude gave me a different perspective. I look at Leibish as a little person, so very helpless and dependent, who affords me endless gratification and fulfillment at every turn.

At this point, Raizy and I are the only ones free to come

home during lunch time and help Mommy with Leibish's feedings. Etty is working uptown, and the boys are in *yeshivah*. I have to admit we are a great help, and it gives us pleasure to know we are lightening her burden somewhat.

Almost the whole day revolves around the baby's feedings. He sleeps an awful lot. It seems to me that if he would not be woken up for his feedings, he would just go on sleeping. I know that might be an exaggeration, but I am sure he does not cry as much as other babies when they are hungry or in pain. Even when he does cry, the sound is much weaker, and the crying much shorter than normal.

I am slowly learning to observe the many differences between Leibish and so called "normal" babies. Almost everything in his little body is somehow different. His head is tiny, almost as if his brain were smaller and needed less room. It is hard to tell where his head and neck meet at the back. There is no indentation at the neck, it is flush with the head. His arms and legs are disproportionately short. His little ears protrude, giving him a special, cute look.

I must admit, even though I know it was wrong of me, that in the beginning when I started to see how different he was, I thought to myself, "This baby is like someone from another world, a stranger, not one of us." Slowly, as I got used to him, I began to accept him as a member of my family and learned to think of him as what he was—a new addition to our family. Altogether, I am beginning to think he is adorable, almost like a little Raggedy Ann, especially when I hold him and he seems as floppy as a rag doll.

I try not to worry, but sometimes I think to myself, "How will he ever learn to do anything? How can he learn new things if all he does is sleep and eat?" It seems as if he was born without any muscles; even his mouth hardly moves. Giving him a bottle is a real challenge and can test the most patient nerves. Now Mommy has started feeding him solids, and that proves even harder. When she puts the spoon into his mouth, he just doesn't seem to know what to do with it. Every feeding takes almost two hours. He falls asleep often during the feedings. I don't blame him. It is as tiring for him as it is for the one feeding him. No wonder the doctor complains he is not gaining enough weight. At his last visit, when he was already five months old, he weighed only eight pounds! Mommy is sick with worry.

I can't get over the fact that the doctor is so quick with his criticism. He acts as if Mommy is not taking proper care of the baby. If the doctor is such a professional, why can't he give her some helpful advice on how to teach little Leibish to eat better? Mommy is afraid to ask or complain about the hard time she is having. She knows he will just look at her with a knowing look and remark, "Well, Mrs. Weinfeld, you know you should have placed him in an institution. I advised you immediately to give him up to experienced people who know how to handle *these* children. Now you see that you can't cope . . ."

So we muddle through the days, coaxing, cajoling. Every spoonful ingested, every ounce swallowed, is a triumph in itself. By the time the feeding is over, it is almost time for the next. Mommy appreciates that we come home during the day; it gives her a little break.

My greatest wonder through all this is that Mommy has still not accepted the fact that Leibish has a big problem, one that he will always live with. Having gone through so much suffering, and having survived it all, gave her superhuman faith that this, too, could be overcome. She insists it is impossible that her little baby is mentally retarded. Although she sees how slow he is to develop and that he looks different from her other children, she believes she must continue to search for the right *shaliach* who can cure him. Every time she hears of a doctor who is big in this field she puts everything on hold and trudges off to his office with Leibish in her arms.

The way I see it, in this day and age, when they are planning to send people to the moon and have come up with computers that can store infinite information, I sure hope more research is done on Down's Syndrome and that our Leibish can still benefit from it in the coming years.

I look at Leibish lying so innocently in his crib, and I think to myself, "How innocent he is. He doesn't realize what upheaval he has brought to this house." Nothing seems the same. Mommy has been affected worst of all. Tatty is away most of the day. He comes home from his daytime job, grabs a bite and is off once again on some catering assignment, but Mommy has not come to terms with herself. She lies in bed a lot, claiming she is tired. I know her better than that. Before Leibish was born, she was a bundle of energy. There was no such thing as laying in bed during the day. I still remember, although I was barely five, how she was up and about almost immediately after Lezer was born. Tatty had to beg her to take a nap in middle of the day so she could make up for the hours she spent rocking little Lezerl during the night.

Now, whenever I come home from school, if she is not busy with Leibish, she can be found lying in bed, staring blankly at the ceiling. She used to enjoy a good book on those rare occasions when she found some respite from her busy schedule. The sewing machine was constantly running, the mixer almost never leaving the counter. Now the sewing machine sits idle, and Mommy just cooks the bare minimum.

She has lost interest in almost everything. It's as if the depression that has engulfed her has a life of its own, holding her in its tenacious grip. There is not much we can do except wait it out and hope that her strong personality will triumph, as it has always done through the hard times in her life.

A Crucial Decision

▼

Wednesday, June 30, 1965

Summer vacation has arrived. The finals are over, and I find I finally have some free time to sit and write about all that transpired these last few months. A lot has happened, and I better write it down before I forget and leave something out.

Right before *Pesach*, Etty got engaged to this tall, handsome young man. The two of them sure make one gorgeous couple. His name is Hershel, and he is from Switzerland. His whole manner speaks of European upbringing. He loves little Leibish and treats him as he would any other little brother-in-law. He throws Leibish up into the air until he touches the ceiling with his little fists and giggles away. He bought us girls lovely necklaces (not as pretty or extravagant as he did for his *kallah*, but we will forgive him this time). For Shloimy and Lezer he got gold necktie pins, and for Leibishl a silver rattle. He is very proper, and we American "roughies" get a kick out of it.

Two weeks after the engagement, my parents invited him

over for the Friday night *seudah*. Raizy and I placed a beautiful tablecloth with matching napkins on the dining room table. We used our silver cutlery, which is set aside for special occasions, and when we were all finished, we took a step back and surveyed our handiwork proudly. Just then, Raizy came up with an idea. Why not place the perforated serving spoon on Hershel's napkin and watch how he goes about eating the soup with it? Surely, his well-bred manners would keep him from protesting that he couldn't possibly eat his soup properly with this "holy" spoon that looked like Swiss cheese.

We could hardly wait for the men to come home. Throughout the *zemiros* we avoided each other's eyes, so that we shouldn't burst out laughing. Finally, it was time for the soup, and we held our breaths as our "Swiss" guest reached for his spoon. To our surprise, we noticed that his spoon had no holes. Did he possess some kind of witchcraft? We were disappointed that our trick did not work and started to eat our portion. This time the joke was on us. It was Raizy who had to go about eating soup with the "holy" spoon. Hershel had switched the spoons while we had gone into the kitchen for the soup plates.

The engagement period passed quickly. *Pesach* came two weeks after the *tenaim*, and the wedding date was set for *Lag B'Omer*, hardly six weeks after the engagement. Hershel's father had come to America for the engagement and expressed his desire to stay till after the wedding, provided it be as soon as possible. Obviously, Hershel's parents are not so well off and cannot afford to travel often. His mother and sisters are not even planning to come. His younger brother, who is learning here in America, will be the only other member of his immediate family to attend the wedding.

Hershel works in the jewelry business and brings home a

nice salary. He even sends his family money every month to help his parents support their large family. His father is frail and cannot work full time.

Everyone decided that the *kallah* must have been a big *nosher*, since it rained throughout the wedding day, right through the night. My parents worried that there would be a very small crowd, but their worries were quickly dispelled as more and more people came, some even uninvited, just to say *mazel tov*. Etty is one of the first from the new generation to get married. A wedding today is a novelty, and people don't want to miss the opportunity to witness this miracle of a new generation rebuilding. Actually, the rain had the opposite effect. It caused everyone to make an extra effort, each thinking, "If everyone will stay home because of the rain, what kind of wedding will the Weinfelds have?"

Tatty catered the affair all by himself so as to cut down on expenses. The sweet table was a masterpiece. There were watermelons in the shape of sail boats, and everything was laid out very artistically. There was loads of food—enough for another wedding—which we were all sure would go to waste. It turned out a fortunate circumstance. The *mesader kidushin* was to be the Skulener Rebbe, newly arrived from Europe, and there would be no *chupah* until he came. Everyone waited and waited; people were becoming impatient as hour followed hour with no Rebbe in sight. Tatty paced back and forth. The guests had to be entertained, and the waiters ran around serving cakes, *hors d'oeuvres* and drinks. I hate to think what would have happened had Tatty not prepared all that extra food.

At eleven-thirty p.m., the Skulener Rebbe finally arrived, as he had been held up by the bad weather. The *chupah* took place on the roof, and everyone climbed up the steep steps. We were all amazed how almost everyone had stayed on despite the late hour. In spite of the delay and the rain, it was a beautiful affair and everyone had a great time.

Someone took movies of the whole wedding. Hershel wants his family should at least get to see the movies, to ease their disappointment at not being able to join at his *simchah*. I can't wait to see the movies after they are developed. Can you imagine? Years from now we will be able to see exactly how everyone moved and danced at this wedding. Next thing you know, they will have sound movies where we will even hear the music and everyone talking.

The proofs are already back from the photographer, and I must admit that we all looked stunning. It is unbelievable how Mommy managed to sew all our dresses in such a short time, a mere six weeks, with *Pesach* still in between. Even Etty's wedding gown was home sewn. No one could believe Mommy had made it. It had yards of fabric, and the skirt had almost a dozen layers of lace. Mommy looked so young, some people thought she was one of the sisters. I'm sure Mommy was pleased, as every woman likes to hear how young she looks. Leibish was left home with a babysitter since he was only eleven months old, and there was no point in bringing him. Perhaps, by the time Shloimy gets married, he will be old enough to come, too.

The first *sheva berachos* was held in the living room, where all our *simchos* take place. Everything was homemade, and the whole house was filled with a delicious aroma. The guests arrived in time and all commented on how beautiful and delicious everything was. This *simchah* has pulled Mommy, somewhat, out of her depression, and she gave it her all.

Little Leibishl was placed in a little port-a-crib in the corner of the living room, the "ladies section." He seemed to be enjoying the singing, as he cooed along contentedly. *Baruch Hashem*, he had eaten quite nicely before the *sheva berachos* began, and Raizy even managed to get some mashed potatoes and apple sauce into him. I wonder if he'll ever learn to eat like a normal child. He hardly gains weight. At eleven months he weighs only eleven pounds three ounces, which is not much more than a newborn. There I go again, can't I put the worries aside for even one day?

While everyone was busy eating and talking and altogether having a good time, I happened to glance in the direction of the crib. I noticed how my two aunts were bending over the baby and looking at each other very secretively. They whispered to each other for a few minutes and then returned to their seats looking very distraught.

I got busy after that with serving dessert and cleaning away. I completely forgot the little incident, until my aunts came over to my parents to take leave at the end of the *sheva berachos*. It seemed unusual for them to wait until everyone left. Normally, they would be the first to leave so they could catch the last bus to Williamsburg. I became curious to see why they stayed so late. Sure enough, Shifra blurted out, "Chaim, I must tell you that I am very hurt."

"But Shifra, I can't imagine what happened. You seemed to be having a good time, and we even made sure to seat you next to cousin Miru. Besides, I am surprised at you. You are not the type to get hurt so easily. What happened, Shifra?"

"Well, Fraidy and I went over to the baby during the *sheva berachos*. We haven't been here for a while, and the last few times we were here the baby was always napping. Once, when he was up, we just saw him for a second before one of your kids yanked him away to another room. Today was the first time we could have a good look at him. And we saw. Oh, Chaim, why didn't you tell us? We feel so bad. You know we love you and would do anything for you. I'm sure we could have helped you and Sara this past year. It must have been so hard on you."

Tatty shifted from one foot to another, very uncomfortable. He was very relieved when Lezer called him from the other room.

"Tatty, where should I put the rented chairs? I folded them all myself.".

He almost ran to Lezer to help out, and somehow, it took him forever to come back. By the time he came back, my aunts had already left, and the subject was closed once again.

I hope that in time my aunts, as well as everyone else in our extended family and in the neighborhood, will come to accept Leibish as part of our family.

As soon as all the *sheva berachos* were over, Mommy started to drift back into her depression. She again showed little interest in her social life and the many activities she had engaged in so enthusiastically in the past. She, who loved sitting up Friday nights till well past midnight to chat and discuss anything and everything, hardly joined in our conversations.

About two week after the *sheva berachos*, and with *Shavuos* behind us, Mommy heard about some famous psychiatrist who was doing research on mongolism. We were dismayed that she would go, her heart full of promise and hope, only to come back totally thwarted with disillusionment when she would see once again that her dearest wish, to have Leibish cured, could not come true. However, there was nothing for us to do except wait it out and see what would happen.

Mommy forewarned us that she might be away for quite a while, perhaps two weeks, and that we would have to stay home in the meantime to fend for ourselves. She had been told that Leibish might be put through extensive and grueling tests to be performed in an out-of-state hospital. She scheduled the appointment for the following Monday morning.

Monday morning saw my parents and Leibish off at seven-thirty a.m. to the office of this newly discovered "great psychiatrist," who would be supervising the tests. They had packed a large suitcase, had borrowed money (the procedure was not covered by our health insurance, and Mommy claimed money was no object when it came to Leibish's welfare), and with their faces set in grim expressions, they were off.

The house suddenly became very quiet. The full impact of their trip started hitting us. Etty was married, and the whole household was left to us young girls. But when we considered that their "trip" was for a great cause, that they had gone to seek the ever elusive help, we did not complain. We packed our lunches and hurried off to school.

When I came back from school, I expected to see all the lights off. I was prepared to enter a dark, empty house—something I dread; I always think there might be some monster lurking under a bed. I gingerly ascended the steps and—lo and behold!—the kitchen light was on. Was Raizy home early today? Had she perhaps skipped the last period to get a head start on supper? Or had someone who did not belong there decide that the light would help him look for what he had come to find?

Suddenly, I heard voices and discerned that they belonged to none other than my parents. But what were they doing home? They weren't due for at least another week or two.

I quickly turned the knob with my key and entered, looking from one parent to the other. Tatty smiled when he saw my puzzled expression.

"I can see you are surprised to see us," he said. "Does that mean you are disappointed that we are back?"

I ran over and planted a kiss on his cheek. "Of course not. I am so happy to have you both home. What happened? Didn't the doctor show up?"

"No, the doctor was there as scheduled," Mommy replied. "We had an interview with him, as is the normal procedure before a patient is to be admitted for testing. I've had many disappointments this past year. The doctors were very negative, and I always ended up leaving their office in tears. They always feel a need to 'reassure' me that Leibish will never learn to read and write, would probably never walk or be trained, and that I'm best off institutionalizing him or finding a suitable foster home so that the rest of the children won't be adversely affected.

"This time I took the initiative and asked the doctor if he could answer some of my questions before we were to proceed. He promised he would try his best to answer as honestly and accurately as possible. First, I asked if the test would harm Leibish in any way. The doctor paused for a minute and then answered uncomfortably. 'I promised to be fair, and so I must tell you that, yes, in most likelihood Leibish will suffer a moderate setback after the two weeks are up. The tests are pretty tough. Many blood samples are drawn, and all kinds of experimental exercises are performed. Glancing at your baby's records, I can see he is very underweight. He weighs less than twelve pounds and is almost a year old. By the time his hospital stay is over, his weight will be even lower, perhaps as low as ten pounds.'

"I felt sick, and I could hear my heart beat wildly inside me. I controlled myself and continued with my questions. I asked what exactly they were testing him for and what the hopes of finding a cure were. Again, the doctor promised to be impartial in his response. 'As you requested,' he said, 'we are to reassess his condition and ascertain if he is indeed a mongoloid. We would then proceed to examine whether it is treatable.'

"There was one question I still had. I knew that this would be the deciding factor. 'Has anyone, to date, been cured of mongolism?'

"The doctor was shocked at my abrupt question. 'I have one answer for you and it consists of one word—no!'

"I looked at Tatty, and he looked at me. We both knew we were taking the next train home, that this was the last time we were going to a psychiatrist. It was up to us to help Leibish. Running from one doctor to another was a waste of time and effort. Obviously, they did not know much more than we did. It was time we pooled our resources and got on with life. And here we are."

Mommy claims that the visit was a worthwhile experience. It has lifted a heavy burden off her shoulders. Ever since Leibish was born, she went back and forth between denying he was a mongoloid and hoping to find a cure for it. This was the only way she could face her child and her life on a daily basis. The thought of knowing he had an irreversible condition was so overwhelming, she just pushed it out of her mind.

Now she has finally come face to face with reality. She must accept that her Leibish is a mongoloid and that, so far, there is no cure for it. She has not given up hope that somewhere down the road a cure might be found to reverse mongolism. But she does not sit and brood about it. Instead, she concentrates on stimulating the baby and making the best of the situation.

Mommy is back to her old self, as if released from an invisible prison. She goes out every day, strolling with Leibish on the avenue, shopping and preparing for the country. Loaves of *kokosh* and marble cakes are produced every Friday, along with delicious *challos*. She joins in at the table, talking and joking along with the rest us.

Tatty is thrilled with the change in her. Even Leibish feels it. He has started to roll over both ways, and his muscles are not nearly as flimsy as they used to be. Mommy has initiated an informal exercise program. Every time she changes his diaper, she spends ten to fifteen minutes bending and stretching his body, flexing his limbs every way possible. She talks and sings to him all the time. Besides enjoying this new game, Leibish has become more active and responsive. She has accomplished more with her iron will these last few weeks, than all the so-called professionals combined. She is full of hope. I am not even surprised; I knew Mommy would come out of it sooner or later, but I'm sure glad it was sooner.

Lezer's Discovery

▼

Wednesday, August 3, 1966

Today I was playing jump-rope with a few of my friends. Lezer was sitting on a bench nearby with his friend Shimi Tauber. While waiting for my turn, I heard them discussing their little brothers. Shimi's brother Dovy is just two weeks younger than Leibish.

"Leibish can crawl already," said Lezer proudly. "And yesterday he even stood alone for a few seconds."

"Big deal," replied Shimi. "Dovy is even younger than him, and he is walking already since *Chanukah*. When he started walking he was eighteen months old, and my mother even said that it was pretty late, compared to the rest of us. I was the fastest," he added, a proud grin on his face. "I started when I was only eleven months old."

"But Leibish speaks already," Lezer said. "My mother says that some children concentrate so much on doing things like walking, that they push off learning other things. I started

47

walking quite early, too, but I didn't start talking until I was over two years old. I bet Leibish speaks even more than I did at his age."

"Yeah, what does he say?" Shimi challenged.

"He says 'Mama' and 'Tata.' And when he wants to go outside he pulls at you and says, 'Ba Ba.'"

"Big deal. Dovy speaks in sentences already. My mother is planning to send him to play school after the *Yamim Tovim* so that she could go back to work."

I could see Lezer deep in thought. I could imagine what was going through his mind. It was out of the question to send Leibish to play school. We all knew that. He had started crawling even later than Dovy was walking. Even the few words Lezer claimed Leibish has mastered need a stretch of the imagination to understand. What Lezer hadn't realized up to now was that there was anything unusual about that. He accepted his little brother as just a regular child. Etty's baby is much younger and still behind Leibish in many ways. Only now did Lezer come face to face with the fact that his brother was different.

My musings came to a short stop.

"Okay, girls who wants to play *J.J. Chalav Yisrael*?" I heard Faigy's loud voice. "The two losers of the last game get to turn the rope."

How generous, I thought bitterly. Faigy somehow is always the one to lead the game, though it's not as if anyone appointed her to this leadership. She just assumes it as naturally as some people inhale oxygen.

One of the "lucky losers" was me, and I became involved with the new game, forgetting the boys' discussion momentarily. I resolved to give Bracha, the notorious champion of

jump rope, a run for her money. No more letting her get away
with, "It's not fair, they were turning too fast, the rope was not
touching the ground." Bad enough that she outjumps and
outplays us in every game, she won't even admit to any of the
few times she is out. (I'm ashamed to admit, but those few times
give me much pleasure—I hope no one notices when I smile
inside while pretending to feel sorry for her. I wonder if the
others feel as I do—that they, too, hope I don't see their "inside
smiles.")

Sure enough, there was no need to hide my inner smile.
There was none. Instead, I had to hide my "inside frown" while
pretending an outside smile. Bracha was the victor once again.

I am learning an important lesson in life. There are losers (in
this case, turners) and there are winners; there are givers and
there are takers; there are followers and there are leaders.
Worrying and fretting will not change the roles. They will only
make the losers (turners), givers and followers into miserable
losers, givers and followers. It's best I learn these things early
and accept my role in life happily and without jealousy.

This evening, I was certain Lezer would bring up the subject
of Leibish and how he was lagging behind his friend's brother.
However, Lezer did not mention anything. Had he forgotten
about it? The look on his face this afternoon did not suggest he
would forget so fast. It seemed to eat at him, and I am sure it gave
him plenty to think about, plenty to ask about. He is usually very
curious and inquisitive, and does not rest till he gets an answer,
even if it means digging and researching to find out for himself.
He did not earn the reputation of "being very smart" for nothing.

I guess he accepts this new revelation as a matter of course.
Besides, I know him well. He'll do anything not to upset my

parents. He probably thinks they don't know and wants to hide it from them. I find it best not to interfere. Let him feel important keeping such a "big secret" all to himself.

Sunday, February 5, 1967

It was after supper. The dishes were washed, the kitchen floor swept. There had been no arguments as to whose turn it was to do what. Conventions were thrown out the window. We must forego our usual meticulous and painstaking demands for fairness and concentrate on finishing as quickly as possible. The risk of getting to wash one more dish or sweep one extra crumb were overlooked for the cause.

Midterms ruled the house. We got down to studying for our midterms with great seriousness. Shloimy, home from the out-of-town *yeshivah* with the flu, looked on indifferently. "A bunch of fanatics," he probably thought to himself, with an aloofness only teenage boys possess. Mommy was at the sewing machine, and Tatty was working late. Little Leibish was occupied somewhere in the house. No one was particularly concerned about him.

Engrossed in her sewing, Mommy obviously forgot the golden rule, "Always check on your child when things are too quiet."

Suddenly, we heard Mommy from the kitchen exclaiming, "Leibish! What did you do?"

We all came rushing into the kitchen. We did not see anything unusual and wondered what was amiss. Moreover, instead of finding Mommy upset, she had a broad smile on her face.

"What happened, Mommy?" we asked, puzzled.

"Leibish broke the new set of china I just bought last month," she replied.

Now we were even more stumped. First, we saw no sign of any broken dishes, and then this business of being almost happy they broke!

"But, Mommy," I said. "I don't see anything broken. And why are you so pleased about all this?"

We knew Mommy did not splurge, and when she did buy something, it was carefully planned and saved for.

"Just open the bottom cabinet under the sink, and you'll find out for yourselves," was all Mommy said.

Lezer, a nimble nine-year-old, always ready to solve a mystery whether real or imagined, was the first to open the cabinet. Sure enough, we saw the broken dishes, each dish piled neatly back in its original place. We had to smile, too.

"Leibish got hold of those dishes and broke them," Mommy went on proudly. "Immediately, he must have realized that this spelled trouble. He then proceeded to pack everything back onto the shelf."

In the meantime, Leibish was sitting in a corner, looking out of the corner of his eyes to see if "the coast was clear." When he realized that Mommy was indeed not angry, he continued playing with his favorite toys, the empty containers Mommy kept for storing leftovers. The rest of us soon forgot the incident.

At the breakfast table the following morning, Mommy announced suddenly, "Wish me good luck, everyone. I am starting to train Leibish."

"But, Mommy," Raizy implored. "Leibish is still too young.

He doesn't even walk yet and says only a few words, very unclearly at that."

We had to admit she was right. Compared to our friends' brothers and sisters who were about the same age, Leibish lagged far behind in most basic skills.

"I am determined, and nothing will change my mind," my mother stated firmly. We all knew that when Mommy spoke in that certain tone, she would not be deterred.

"What made you decide now?" Shloimy asked.

"You may have already forgotten last night's broken dishes," she declared. "To you it might not have held any special significance. However, to me it was a revelation. It proved to me that Leibish was far more intelligent than I thought. If he had the sense to cover up his act, something even normal children would not do at the young age of two-and-a-half years, then I am confident that he is smart enough to be trained."

The next two weeks were busy ones for Mommy. Mommy did not bake or sew (a very rare event), concentrating completely on her grand task. Admittedly, it was very difficult. Any mother of perfectly healthy children will tell you that one of the hardest jobs with little children is getting them to stay clean. I see from my friends' little siblings how many hours and days their mothers sit there—not always so patiently, mind you—trying to stop their little kid from irrigating the carpet for the umpteenth time. Just the other day, I was visiting Rifky Schneider when we both burst out laughing. Her little brother Zevi was happily waving to his father from the window as he was leaving for *Minchah*. Even when his father was already out of sight, Zevi continued waving, completely unaware of having soaked up the couch in the process.

Mommy, being a very busy woman, did not waste time studying books on so-called "Modern Parenting." Shlomo Hamelech writes in *Koheles*, "He who holds back the rod hates his son." The first time Leibish had an accident, she gently tried to show him that it was wrong, as she usually did when guiding him through new habits. When this proved useless, she did not give up. A little spanking on the seat would be a small price to pay for such a great step they were embarking on. When she gave him a gentle little spanking, Leibish cried somewhat, but he immediately stopped when he accomplished his first "sitting" on the potty successfully. When two weeks were up, Mommy proclaimed victory. We had a hard time deciding who was prouder, Leibish or Mommy. He clapped his little hands together in delight with a big smile on his face. Everyone cheered.

When Mommy told our family doctor of Leibish's latest achievement, he thought it almost a miracle. He said he would not be surprised if Leibish broke a record, by being the youngest "mongoloid" child to have been trained.

Mommy was horrified to hear that most of the children affected by mongolism who are raised in institutions grow into adulthood without being able to keep themselves "clean." At the same time, though, Mommy felt a glow of pride and admitted to herself that there was nothing like a little determination to get a job done.

What the doctor did not know was that a loving spanking on the little seat was sometimes far more beneficial than all the psychiatric gibberish. It wasn't so long ago that she saw Dr. Maruk, a renowned psychiatrist in Queens who specialized in children like Leibish. She came home from that visit completely shattered. He warned her not to expect much from her little son.

According to statistics, he would probably be trained very late, and possibly grow up into adulthood untrained. His speech would be very limited, and she "shouldn't even dream of him learning to read or write." He went on to warn her that she should never use any physical punishment or scold him, as it would be too traumatic for such a child. The best thing would be to let him live within his own limitations, so long as he remained happy. "Very happy, indeed," Mommy had thought grimly. "Growing up like a little animal would make him very *unhappy*." That visit, too, was a blessing in disguise. Nothing in life ever happens without a purpose, even when at the time it seems pointless. She realized now that it brought out an inner strength and determination she did know she possessed. So much for Dr. Maruk's and the other psychiatrists' high flung ideas.

A Discouraging Experience

▼

Today is the first day of *Pesach* vacation. I don't think we'll ever get finished. During the year, I complain about the shortage of closets and drawers to put all my things in, but come *erev Pesach*, I feel I could do very well with even less space. Wouldn't it be easier if we just lived in one room like they did back in the old days? They didn't even have any carpets to vacuum or linoleums to wax. I sigh with regret just at the thought. Why couldn't I have been born then?

Leibish is not making things any easier. He crawls all over the place and empties the drawers and cabinets constantly.

I asked Mommy, "Why did you take Leibish out of kindergarten? I thought you said that the Sovoyer Rebbetzin is a wonderful lady, and with all the help she has from her volunteers, she would do a great job with Leibish. You even thought it would be good for Leibish to play with normal children."

The pained look on Mommy's face made me stop short.

"Oh no, here I go again," I thought to myself dejectedly. It seems that when the subject is Leibish I always put my foot in my mouth. "I'm sorry, Mommy. I really didn't mean to upset you."

"You have every right to ask," she said. "I'm sure you are also disappointed that Leibish stopped going to kindergarten. It made things easier on all of us, and it seemed like a good idea. The Sovoyer Rebbetzin welcomed Leibish into her little school and promised to make every effort to keep him in spite of his disability. I didn't worry much. 'What can happen in kindergarten?' I thought. 'The children just run around and spend the day in free play, eating lunch and some singing.' I was confident it would work out. Besides, I was encouraged by Leibish's progress. He hasn't had an accident in weeks. He knows to point to the potty and say, 'Uh, uh.' Even though he doesn't walk, we just have to lead him by the hands and 'mission accomplished.'" Mommy sighed. "Tatty started having doubts about the whole idea. When he went after a few days to see how Leibish was doing, he was dismayed to see how wild and overactive he was. At home, Leibish already knows the rules of the house, more or less, and is manageable most of the time. However, at the kindergarten, Leibish was so excited with all the toys and children that he became disruptive. He didn't know quite what to make of his new surroundings. His behavior was less than acceptable. He threw blocks at his playmates and pushed trucks into anyone in his way. The children seemed scared to go near him. Things were getting out of hand. Tatty didn't say anything and hoped that maybe he was exaggerating things to himself.

"Yesterday, sure enough, the *rebbetzin* called, and I knew right away there was trouble. 'Hello, I am sorry to call with bad news,' she said, 'but I have to tell you that my kindergarten is really not suitable for Leibish.'

"It was as if she'd thrown a rock at me. 'He is very sweet, but much too wild,' she continued. 'He is destroying toys and disrupting the group. Maybe we'll try again next year, when he is a little older.'"

"Were you very hurt, Mommy?" I asked.

"Of course, I was. Knowing his shortcomings still doesn't stop me from being hurt when I come face to face with the hard facts. On the other hand, even though it may hurt, I realize now, two-and-a-half long and precious years later, that the only way to manage with a special child is to look reality in the face and tell yourself that this is it; you can't change things, but you can change yourself. By persistence and hope, you can endure the disappointments that come your way. I just have to keep my eyes open and see the positive.

"The fact is, since Leibish has entered our lives, everything seems to have turned around for the better. Of course, things were all right before, too. Since Leibish was born, however, things have become even better. We have never done so well financially as we do now. Leibish has brought a special *berachah*, and whatever ventures we start thrive as never before. Etty has done a wonderful *shidduch*, and I myself have become a better and happier person. I have my priorities straighter and know to thank Hashem for the little things in life, things I used to take for granted."

I should have known Mommy's answer. She never tired of telling us, as well as herself, that she believed firmly in "looking up to see how good it *will* be and looking down to see how bad it *could have* been."

Upsherin

▼

Monday, August 7, 1967

Tatty came up from the city early last week. When I came back from my morning swim on Wednesday, he was already sitting at the kitchen table in our bungalow sipping a glass of ice-cold seltzer. (Tatty always says, "Something that should be served cold should be *very cold*, while something that should be served hot should be *very hot*.") Usually, he comes up Thursday evenings, still earlier than most of the other men in our colony. (The trip up from the city sometimes takes as long as four hours. There are very narrow roads, many unpaved, with few lanes. When there is traffic on the weekends, it could be bumper-to-bumper most of the way.) But last week Tatty came even earlier. After all, it was Leibish's *upsherin*.

For some reason, Leibish's hair did not grow as long or as thick as my other brothers' did at this age. I saw a picture of Shloimy right before his haircut, and I could tell he had a full head of hair reaching down to his waist. Lezer, too, had very

58

long hair. There is no need to look at any pictures of Lezer. It was only seven years ago, and I still remember what he looked like. Everyone used to comment, "What a beautiful little girl! And such long hair!"

I am noticing that altogether everything about Leibish is on the slow side; his learning as well as his physical growth are delayed. None of my friends in the country believed he was already three years old, and that he was getting his haircut this week. Now that they see he has little *payos* and that he wears *tzitzis*, they admit that I wasn't just making it all up. I don't blame them, though. If I didn't know better, I would have guessed his age at no more than two. Aside for the fact that he doesn't wear diapers—which not everyone notices, and no one would go over to him and check if he indeed does not wear any—he doesn't do anything more than a two-year-old. He is even shorter than some other two-year-old toddlers I see around this bungalow colony.

Admittedly, I am proud of him, nonetheless. When we asked him before his haircut what he was going to get, he said, "*Payos* and *tzitzis*." At night, when we start saying *Shema* with him, he shakes his head vigorously; he understands that it means his bedtime and lets us know that he is vehemently against it. When he gets up in the morning and his diaper is dry, he says, "*Triken vi feffer*" (a Yiddish expression meaning very dry; literally, "as dry as pepper"). To an outsider, his speech is completely unintelligible, but we are slowly learning to understand.

I'm sure Mommy is not as excited as by her other sons. At a time like this, when Leibish reaches another milestone, there are mixed feelings. On the one hand, we are happy to see him grow up and do things like normal children. Having *payos* and *tzitzis* make him look just like other three-year-olds. However, the similarities end there. Whereas other boys go with their fathers to a first grade in a *cheder* and say the *aleph-bais* with the *rebbe* while the class gets *pekelech*, Leibish did none of these things. There was no point in taking him to a class full of mischievous boys, who would immediately notice something different in Leibish and would probably make fun of him, or at least sit there and stare, making everyone present very uncomfortable. Besides, Leibish does not understand what this is all about and would not cooperate.

My parents think it best to keep everything on a small scale, as quiet as possible. That does not mean that they hide Leibish or are ashamed of being with him in public. Quite the contrary, they take him everywhere they go, to family *simchos* and whenever they go visiting. They just don't feel it is necessary to draw needless attention to him and cause unnecessary unpleasantness to our family. People can be very ignorant and thoughtless. They can come over to my parents and try to console them at a time when parents should be congratulated. Or they can pretend that all is normal with Leibish and say something like, "May he grow up to be a *talmid chacham*." Over the last three years, I have heard enough such talk, and I see no reason to invite more of it.

Right before the summer, when Mommy was sitting with Leibish in her dress shop, reading a story to him, a customer walked in. The customer looked at Leibish and then at Mommy. Mommy could tell she wanted to say something. The normal thing to have said at such a time would have been something like, "Oh, that's such a nice thing to do. Not too many mothers would sit in middle of the day and read stories to their children." Instead, she was dismayed when the woman grimaced and said in a very unpleasant manner, "Mrs. Weinfeld, don't you think it would be a good idea to place this child in a home? You know he won't amount to anything, so why risk it?"

When my mother, who was already very upset, asked her what she meant by risking it, the woman warned, "You know very well this child can cause trouble when you will want to marry off your other children."

"But I already married off my eldest daughter to a fine young man after Leibish was born."

"Mrs. Weinfeld, just because your foolishness succeeded once does not mean you can get away with it a second time," the insensitive woman continued.

My mother picked up Leibish who was sitting on the chair, happily licking a lollypop, oblivious to this evil woman's opinion of him. She ran to the dressing room in the back of the store and cried her heart out. She held her little boy against her bosom, as if protecting him from this wicked woman, who no doubt felt very noble by offering her generous advice to this "foolish" mother.

Mommy is as familiar with crying as some people are with breathing. It takes very little to set her off. Why couldn't people just be quiet and keep their insensitive opinions to themselves? Why couldn't they learn from the others who are so kind and accepting of Leibish, and who always let us know that they are ready to help us out whenever necessary?

Turning Point

▼

Thursday, September 14, 1967

Today is Sunday, my favorite weekday. There is school until twelve o'clock, after which I come home and am free to do anything I want. Well, not exactly. There is homework, but that can always wait. Somehow, if I don't do it, it waits patiently for me. Besides, there are chores to attend to and errands to run.

Today is no exception, and I am off to Martin Paint to get Mommy paint for another coat she is planning to apply to our woodwork, in time for the *Yamim Tovim*.

I don't have to be told where Martin Paint is. It's been there for as long as I remember. Somehow, certain stores just stay there, comforting in their constancy. "If only these stores would be closed on *Shabbos*," I thought with irritation. "It's about time the non-Jewish store owners recognized that we are a majority in the neighborhood. They should respect our holidays." But then, I had to admit that there are many Jewish stores now, and walking in Boro Park on *Shabbos* has become a pleasure.

62

I took Leibish along. There was no other way. Neither I nor Raizy ever leave the house without Leibish. My friends have learned to accept him as part of the scenery. I count myself truly blessed with such nice friends. They just act as if he is normal. With his sweet smile and lively manner, I am certain that they feel genuinely charmed by him. Leibish is always happy to go "bye bye." Although he is already over three years old, he doesn't walk yet, so I placed him in the stroller and off we went.

When I arrived at the store, I made sure to act as quickly as possible. "The less I exposed Leibish to new people," I reasoned, "the better." I hated being asked about him, and even worse, when they didn't ask and just stared in that peculiar way. As I turned to leave, Leibish slipped himself out of the stroller and started towards the center of the store. Instinctively, I grabbed him and almost threw him back in the stroller.

"Leibish, let's go!" I was almost frantic.

"It is not his fault to have been born that way," a kind voice called out.

I turned around to see who had said that and realized it was the owner himself. G-d bless him! He has freed me. A new world has opened for me. I will never, ever be ashamed of him again. Instead, I will love him even more and be proud of his slow but steady progress and applaud his many accomplishments.

October, 1967

Leibish is walking! To me it is a miracle. All the hard work of the past months have finally paid off.

It seemed almost hopeless. Every time we walked him across the room and let go of him, he would plop right down. Lately, he seemed pretty ready to walk on his own. His balance was excellent, and we felt he only held on to us for fear of letting go and falling. Well, he did it, and we are so happy.

A few days ago, Raizy was walking Leibish across our front porch. It was a mild day, and she figured Leibish would not protest as much as he did sometimes in the house when participating in this exercise. Sometimes, when I see his reluctance to exert himself in some physical activity, I think he is lazy. Shloimy theorizes that it has something to do with his mental state. A normal child wants to learn new activities to keep up with the older children and adults around him. It gives him the ambition to try again and again, even when things are hard to master. Leibish, on the other hand, does not have this intellectual reasoning. He is laid back and content. He sees no reason to exert himself to reach higher planes. Therefore, he must be given extra incentive and stimuli to achieve the basic milestones normal children accomplish on their own.

Raizy has a lot of patience and doesn't give up easily. So many times, Leibish refused to go on with the walking lesson. Who can blame him? These lessons had been going on for over a year, since he learned to stand while holding on, and he got frustrated and bored. He balked when taken away from his favorite corner, where he'd sit quietly with his matchbox cars. Raizy would plant a lollypop at the other end to make him press on just a little longer.

On that momentous afternoon, Leibish, led by Raizy, walked sturdily across the porch. When Raizy hesitatingly let go of him, he remained standing on his own. To Raizy's amazement, he started walking alone, haltingly at first and then more firmly with each new step. She grabbed Leibish and showered him with at least a hundred kisses. She ran into the house, straight to the sewing machine.

"Mommy, you won't believe it," she shouted. "Leibish is walking by himself!"

Without answering, Mommy ran to the phone and dialed a number.

"Chaim, I have great news. Leibish is finally walking!"

We all stood there with big smiles on our faces and shared this precious moment together. Only a family with a special child can know the extraordinary joy that comes at such times.

What a relief it is to have Leibish walk at last. It was a very awkward feeling to have a boy well over three years old crawling all over the place. It seemed very unnatural and uncomfortable. Imagine how heavy he was to carry around, up and down the stairs and in and out of the carriage. Luckily, we live on the first floor. See, there is always a bright side.

It is a pity that I cannot boast to my friends. My friends are always coming to school, bragging about their brainy little siblings.

"My brother started walking at ten months."

"My sister says fifteen words already, and she is only thirteen months old. The doctor says she is very advanced."

What am I supposed to brag about? Should I have announced last year, "Leibish can hold a spoon, and he is only two and a half"? Or "My brother started saying *hami* (Yiddish baby talk meaning food), and he is only three years old"? If I tell them how excited we all are that Leibish is walking, surely they will ask me how old he is, and then when I tell them, they will giggle and snicker, "Ha, ha. Your brother is a genius, he is already walking at such a young age." Not everyone in my class is as sensitive about Leibish's condition as my close friends are.

I observed almost from the start that this diary is more Leibish's than mine. It proves what a strong influence his presence in our family has on me, and for that matter on the whole family. It's sure lucky that I started this diary the same day Mommy let us know about the impending birth. How *bashert* it was that those two events coincided. If this diary is about Leibish, so be it. I feel honored to record it.

Now that I'm in ninth grade, much of our learning is done through class discussions. We have very interesting philosophical lessons as we learn Jewish history and encounter our great forefathers and their heroic deeds.

Rabbi Gansfried is our history teacher who throughout the year points out the various *gedolim* of yesteryear. We admire them and sigh, "How we wish we could be even somewhat like them!"

Rabbi Gansfried repeatedly emphasizes the importance of achieving our full potential. "Everyone can be like Moshe Rabbeinu!" he proclaims emotionally.

All of us ask, "How can we be like Moshe, the greatest amongst men? Wouldn't it be enough just to be a good Jewish girl?"

"Anyone who reaches his full capacity," Rabbi Gansfried explains, "and utilizes all the talents and intellect he was endowed with by Hashem, is considered to have reached the same heights as Moshe Rabbeinu, who actually achieved his full potential."

In my humble opinion, Leibish could also be considered on that high level. By learning and developing to the best of his ability, by observing *mitzvos* and learning to help others, he will have reached the same heights as the great *gedolei hador*. It is not for us to decide who is great or who has more importance. We are all Hashem's creations, and each of us was put here for a reason.

Once, Rabbi Gansfried tried to test us to see if we got his message. He asked, "I will ask you a question but you must promise to answer truthfully. When you see a beggar on the street, his clothes tattered, his face unwashed and his general demeanor unkempt, do you involuntarily frown and turn away in disgust? Do you subconsciously think to yourself, 'Is there anything positive this unpleasant person can contribute to society? He is dirty, lives like a parasite and altogether is like a thorn in my eyes'? Do you walk away, feeling very smug about your noble bearing and believing yourselves much superior?"

Our silence conveyed our answer. None of us could raise our hands and attest to the contrary. We all had at least one yes to his disquieting questions. We felt annoyed at being made to face this unpleasant fact. Everyone likes to hear how great he is, and no one likes to be made to come face to face with his shortcomings. I guess we are in high school for a purpose. It is time to grow up and learn to overcome our childish notions.

Rabbi Gansfried continued, as if to confirm my thoughts, "You are approaching adulthood, and it is time to change your way of thinking and remember that this 'unappealing beggar' was once a little baby, cute and cuddly, loving and cheerful. He was given a *neshamah*, just like we all were. He wanted the best for himself, just like everybody else. Fate had other things in store for him. Perhaps his parents died, leaving him an orphan without family or financial support. Or perhaps he even grew up in a stable comfortable home, full of love and care. He could even have gone to school, had many friends and been an A student.

"That 'nudgy' lady, let's call her Chana. She stands on the corner begging for 'something for *Shabbos*.' She has a dirty face, with a foolish grin adding to her peculiarity. This same Chana might even have sat in this very classroom. Then, unfortunately, she had a nervous breakdown, *lo aleinu*. Her nerves were weak; they could not take the pressures of growing up and gave way. Can you imagine her family's pain?

"Or take the mother who looked forward so much to having a healthy baby and then was told that her child has a mental illness. Is it possible to measure the enormity of her sorrow?" (Here, I squirmed.) "Some people have weak muscles, some are short, others frail. No one would think to blame them or ridicule them for these weaknesses, because they are so obviously not the person's fault. When we see a poor, demented person, our instinct is to say, 'Oh, I'm sure he could help himself. He is lazy and would rather stand on the street begging for *my* hard-earned money.' When we come across someone who acts bizarre and mad, we laugh and think, 'What a crazy person!' We must look at this mental weakness just the same as we look at a physical weakness. None are anybody's fault, and we must be especially kind to them. Who is to tell which of us is truly great or whose *neshamah* is nobler? In the eyes of Hashem, we are all His special children, and he loves us equally."

I feel fortunate to have fabulous teachers like our Rabbi Gansfried. He surely wouldn't snicker if I would tell him of Leibish's latest accomplishments.

HASC

▼

Tuesday, November 7, 1967

This *Shabbos*, my mother came home with some good news.
She told her friend Mrs. Fishbeyn at *shul* about her search for a
kindergarten for Leibish. She did not elaborate on his special
needs. My parents take it for granted that people know about his
handicaps and see no reason to discuss it with anyone. I have
never yet heard them telling anyone how hard it is on them, or
even sharing his shortcomings with anyone. It seems almost as
if they feel that if they won't talk about it, it will be as if there
is nothing to talk about.

Mrs. Fishbeyn knew how my mother felt about the subject
and did not ask what kind of school she was looking for.
Obviously, Leibish needed a school with special facilities, and
there was no point in pressing the issue. Besides, Mrs. Fishbeyn
herself had a mentally disabled child who was enrolled in
HASC (Hebrew Academy for Special Children) located right
here in Boro Park. She told Mommy that she is very happy with

the school. The children are stimulated, and even learn to read and write. They no longer need to attend *goyishe* schools where they have no contact with *Yiddishkeit*. They have special classes where they learn to master the Hebrew alphabet, learn to make *berachos* and understand the concept of *kashrus*. When they are older, many of the children can *daven* fluently from a *siddur*.

To us, this is more than we had dared hope. Leibish growing up to *daven* just like everyone else? We even went so far as to believe that some day, after his *bar-mitzvah*, he too would be counted in a *mezuman* and a *minyan* in *shul*. In short, *a mensch vee alle menschen*. Tatty agreed it would be a good idea to contact the principal, Rabbi Kahn, right after *Shabbos* and ask for an interview.

The rest of the *Shabbos* passed in great anticipation. A new door has opened for us. Visions of Leibish attending classes for the disabled held at the local public schools used to dance before our eyes, shutting out any hope for Leibish to be educated in a Jewish atmosphere.

I have a hunch that things will improve dramatically from now on. Mommy will be able to breathe more easily knowing that a big load has been lifted off her shoulders. She will have more time to herself and will hopefully learn to relax and enjoy life once more.

December, 1967

Leibish has been attending school for over a month now, and it turned out even better than expected. He is delighted when the van comes to pick him up. There have been some difficulties with the new language he must learn. At home, we speak strictly Yiddish, and in school it is English, of course. HASC is a government-subsidized organization, and they must comply with its rules of being interracial. There are some non-Jewish children, including blacks. It is a disconcerting factor, but I don't think it will have any ill effects on Leibish. The only thing, I am worried about is that some of those children have had very little stimulation and are very behind. We worried that learning a new language, when he has not even mastered the old, would be very confusing to Leibish and would add to his learning disabilities. When Mommy met his new teacher, she was reassured. He is a *frum* young man and speaks Yiddish fluently. He promised he would do his best to ease Leibish slowly into English.

The first day of *Chanukah* vacation, Raizy and I attended a music class held for Leibish's group. The school had invited all the mothers to come observe their children so they could get a closer look at the daily activities at school. Mommy had no one to mind the shop, so she let us go instead.

For us, it was a treat. We were always wondering how the school got Leibish to do things we could not get him to learn, no matter how much we tried. He has learned to speak much better and more clearly and knows to pick up toys after himself. He has learned to share with his niece when Etty comes to visit. He can even put his coat on. He mutters, "Flick flack," as he puts his coat on the floor. He places his hands into the sleeves, and "wham," on it flies, over his shoulders. It usually lands upside down, and he wonders why the hood ends up between his legs. But when he sees that his fingers are actually showing through the sleeves, he smiles proudly. So what if the hood is on the bottom; that is the manufacturer's fault. Now we had the opportunity to get a glimpse of the techniques used with these special children.

We were enchanted by the program and now comprehend why Leibish loves school so much. The music teacher's name is Louise, and she has a sweet soprano voice. She plays the guitar, accompanied by a little drum, and sometimes she switches to the accordian. At her side is an oversized drum, upside down, which serves as a large container for the many instruments used by the kids. First comes the introductory song with a very catchy tune. We still hum it to ourselves all the time.

"Leibish came to school today, Leibish, Leibish,
Leibish came to school today, let's all say Hi!"

And all the little ones chant, "Hi, hi."

In this way, everyone gets to learn each other's name, to greet each other, use some verbal skills, all while having a great time through something they all have in common—a love for music.

There was one little boy, Elchanan by name, who touched everyone's heart. He was the first to respond to the teacher's questions and was very co-operative. He is a very high function-ing little four-year-old, who has already mastered quite a few words and, according to his mother, has been walking since age two-and-a-half. I could see his mother is still very young. In fact, I wouldn't be surprised if he is her first child. Looking at her, no one would believe she had been struck by "tragedy." She apparently loves Elchanan very much and has put a lot of work into him. I am learning that stimulation is the key word with children like Leibish and Elchanan, and that HASC is the place where they could thrive best.

After the introduction, Louise's assistant passes around the large drum. Everyone gets to choose the instrument he or she likes best. Leibish picked a small drum. Elchanan picked a large rattle. Everyone got something else, and the large drum, with some remaining pieces, was returned to its place. Louise then invited each member individually to play his instrument. When it came to Leibish's turn, he could not make any sound come out. He shook and banged the drum but nothing happened. He had no idea that he had to take the little stick attached to it and bang on the drum to produce sound. I ventured to suggest to Louise that perhaps I could give Leibish another instrument which would be easier for him to handle. Louise objected very gently and explained that part of this program is to teach the child to accept the consequences of his actions. This way, he will learn to deal with his mistakes and avoid them in the future. I felt bad for Leibish. He looked very disappointed as he watched how everyone shook their little instruments, and how delighted they were at the sounds and "music" they were producing all on their own.

We were happy when Louise called it quits and announced that it was time for the final part of this lesson. Again, the oversized drum was passed around, and everyone had to return their choices. I waited to see if anyone would refuse to give theirs up, just as Leibish always did when asked to share his toys with Etty's children. No one did. Obviously, they were learning an awful lot here, and sharing was one of the things they were taught.

Then came the best treat of all. All the children were invited to join Louise in playing her guitar. They all pulled and banged at the strings, while Louise herself played as loudly as possible to give it some semblance of a tune. The sound effects were for the birds, but to the children it was music *par excellence*. Their eyes were shining with pure bliss.

We were filled with joy as we watched the children enjoying themselves. Here they were not "*nebechs*" or "retards." They were part of a class, each an individual who could learn and enjoy himself just like anyone else. G-d bless the Kahns (Rabbi Kahn is the founder of HASC) and people like them who have finally started to do something for the countless children with various disabilities, who have until recently had little or no opportunity for advancement. They are finally being integrated into our community and society in general by exposing them to the everyday joys of living.

Leibish to the Rescue

▼

Wednesday, February 5, 1968

Yesterday was our last day of mid-winter vacation, and we had made up with our neighbor, Gitty, to go shopping uptown. Just as we were about to leave, Gitty called to say that she was running a fever and could not come with us. We decided it would be no fun going shopping with only the two of us. Besides, choosing a new skirt was not as simple as all that. When you are fifteen and seventeen (yes, believe it or not, Raizy is already seventeen years old, a *"kalla moid,"* as Mommy's friends like to say), you want to look just so, and at least two opinions besides your own are necessary to assure the proper selection. So we decided to forego shopping and go to Prospect Park instead. With mid-winter vacation going on at many of the other *frum* schools in Brooklyn, we were sure that there would be plenty of Jewish girls around.

We told Mommy of our changed plans, and she was all for us going there to enjoy our last day of vacation. Leibish was in

75

school, and it was one of those rare occasions when we did not feel an obligation to take him along with us. We never minded taking him along, but let's face it, it is still not the same when we have to coax him along every few minutes. We do become impatient when we have to catch a bus and have to remind him to hurry up. I know he can't help himself, that at almost four years old he still walks as slowly and as unsteadily as a two-year-old toddler, but the fact is that it's still easier without him.

When we arrived at the park, it was already full of people. Mothers were there with their pre-schoolers and nannies with their charges. Just as we expected, there were many other girls like us who had come to enjoy winter's pleasures. There was snow on the ground, and we had great fun with our rented sleds making our way down the many hills and slopes.

In time, we got bored and started looking around for some other form of entertainment. Our eyes fell on the lake nearby, and Raizy and I, along with some friends we had met during the course of the morning, decided to "ice-skate" across it. We did notice that no one else had thought of doing it—the lake was empty—but we weren't fazed. Too bad on everyone else who didn't think of this wonderful idea. It was just another proof of our superior intelligence.

We were wearing sturdy, rubber-soled boots, and as we started across the icy waters, we felt there was nothing more exciting than sliding on such a large expanse of ice. We were surely ready to compete in the Winter Olympics.

Suddenly, Raizy let out a shriek. We were horrified when we saw that she had started to sink into the lake. The ice was breaking under her weight. The lake was obviously not as solidly frozen as we had thought. All those people out there were not as dumb, after all. They had been aware of the warm weather we had had the previous few weeks and that the ice was only surface ice formed over the last few days when the weather had suddenly turned cold. But there was no time to think. We started to pull Raizy out of the water. Fortunately, we were still over the shallow parts, and by wading through the now exposed water, we were able to make it to land safely. But not before we had all become drenched to our waists. We were chilled to the bone, and our clothes were dripping with water which was slowly turning into icicles.

We made our way home as quickly as possible. As we neared our house, we were shivering uncontrollably. It was hard to tell whether it was due to our "wet" attire or from our fear that Mommy should find out.

It's a funny thing, this fear of upsetting our parents. I don't remember the last time we got beaten, or even yelled at. And yet we are in terror of getting them angry. It must be that guilt has found its way into the depths of our souls and settled in for good. The guilt of adding to their troubles. The guilt of placing another little pebble in their way back from the despair and hopelessness that not so long ago had engulfed them upon Leibish's birth. It has long been my opinion that Leibish has made things easier for my parents in many ways. It might sound as some kind of joke, but I am quite serious. I am aware of the hardships and the challenges that are involved in raising him, but I also observe that ever since he was born our behavior has improved tremendously. None of us are too *farshlafen* and getting into trouble at school or at home had been a frequent occurrence. After Leibish was born, however, our attitudes changed, and we no longer felt the need to stir up trouble in order to have "fun."

We opened the door. Luckily, the inside lock was open, and all we had to do was turn the key in the door knob and we were inside. We surveyed the kitchen and the room beyond and were relieved to see that no one was there. From the back room came the loud rhythmic sound of the sewing machine. Mommy was hard at work on some new garment and did not hear us entering the house. We made our way down the side steps, leading from the hallway, and in a minute we were downstairs in the large, unfinished basement. Our luck was still holding. Mommy had done the laundry the night before, and all our clothing was hanging neatly across the clothesline. In no time, we were dressed in dry clothes, with the wet ones in place where the dry ones had been. We returned upstairs and came into the room where Mommy was still busy sewing as if nothing was amiss.

Mommy turned around to ask how we had enjoyed ourselves and at once noticed the inevitable. Her sharp eye had discerned that we looked different from when we left. We never learn. Mommy always warns us, "You can't hide anything from a mother." Well, we braced ourselves for the worst and were about to reveal our little piece of mischief, when . . .

"Oh, I hear Leibish's van beeping," Mommy called out. "Will you go and take him off the van? It is slippery out there, and you had better hold him by both hands so he doesn't fall."

We ran like the wind. Little Leibish had arrived to save us just in the nick of time. Never had we been so happy to have Leibish back home from school.

By the time we were back inside, having helped Leibish out of his hat and coat, Mommy seemed to have forgotten the whole episode. Whether she just pretended to, having decided to let us get away with it this time, or had forgotten, we will never know. Neither are we in any mood to find out. It's not worth the risk.

Winter News

▼

Motzai Shabbos, February 22, 1969

Mommy always believed in early stimulation. She claims she can "awaken" those brain cells which are not functioning by exercising them. As Leibish grows up, we see that, indeed, her efforts are bearing fruit. He has learned an awful lot since that day he came into the world and sent everyone's emotions on a roller coaster ride. Not only had Mommy kept him at home and treated him like any other child, she had done much more and continues to feel an obligation to keep on doing, even though Leibish gets to participate in special workouts at school, which help strengthen his gross motor skills (such as sitting and walking) and toughen up his lax muscles. Still, at bath time and while dressing him in the morning and undressing him at night, she tries at every opportunity to keep his muscles in motion. Although he enjoys just sitting in his crib and playing quietly with some toys, she always feels guilty that he is not being stimulated enough.

One *Shabbos*, we were at Bnos as usual, and my parents
were trying to catch a nap. Usually, Leibish would nap, too, and
there was no problem about what to do with him. That particular
Shabbos, Leibish showed no signs of tiredness and stayed
awake. All the lullabies were to no avail. Mommy finally placed
a basket with toys in his crib and went off to her bedroom for
some much needed rest. She could not fall asleep. Her conscience kept bothering her. She tossed and turned. "I shouldn't
just leave him there by himself," she kept thinking. She knew it
was a normal thing to do with a child on a *Shabbos* afternoon
when there was no one around to watch him, and the parents
wanted to sleep, but with Leibish being the way he was, there
was always that fear and guilt that maybe he wasn't being
treated properly.

Sunday, March 2, 1969

This year has been uneventful—no weddings, no *bar-
mitzvahs*, no graduations, no babies. Etty has a growing family;
her third child was born at the end of last year. Raizy is in twelfth
grade and I the tenth. Leibish is in the second year in HASC. The
house has settled into a pleasant routine. Mommy is as busy as
ever juggling the house and her shop. Now that we are older, we
help her a lot with the chores. Come Friday, when she returns
home just two hours before *Shabbos*, the house is spotless, the
table set and the *blech* ready. Leibish is freshly bathed and
dressed in his sailor outfit (that Mommy sewed, of course). We
girls are showered and dressed in our *Shabbos* robes (yes, you

guessed again, that Mommy sewed, of course) and the "big boys," Shloimy and Lezer, are in their *Shabbos* suits in the living room preparing a *Dvar Torah* for the *Shabbos tisch.*

It is hard for me to imagine that it was ever different. There is an aura of peace and happiness that pervades our home. No wonder Mommy claims that Leibish has brought *mazel* into the house. Tatty is planning to give up the catering business, because he claims the store Mommy bought shortly after Leibish was born is bringing in enough money so that he will soon be able to keep only one job. This financial improvement has lessened my parents' tension enormously and has contributed to this calm and tranquility.

We can thus concentrate on our cute, adorable, delicious little Leibishl and observe his own unique personality as it blossoms and unfolds. Although his vocabulary is still very limited, and he speaks only in single words, he has a special talent in expressing himself.

Thursday, March 6, 1969

Etty asked me to come over on Sunday to babysit for her while she goes to a party. I gladly accepted, being that I felt it a treat to spend some time with my wonderful niece and nephews. I took Leibish along and plunged into my responsibilities with gusto. As the hours passed, however, much of the "gusto" vanished. With each glass of milk spilt and the baby crying non-stop, my enthusiasm turned into apathy. I resorted to yelling and screaming. "If you spill your milk one more time,

I'll . . . !" and, "Baby, if you don't stop crying I'll hit the roof!" Had Etty walked in then, it would have been the end of my babysitting career.

Leibish did not help the situation. He wanted a lolly, and when I refused to give him—it was close to suppertime and his appetite is poor as it is—he threw a tantrum and began strewing toys all over the house, adding to the ruckus. The noise level reached a crescendo, and I blew a fit.

My face must have looked quite scary, for out of the corner of my eye I noticed that Leibish, who had been crying and screaming, lay down suddenly on the floor and got very quiet. I came over to see what had happened, whether he had hurt himself and fainted. All the wind went out of me as I saw him close his eyes and pretend to sleep. He had realized I was upset and figured that if I thought he was sleeping, I would not be angry with him. He had guessed right.

Monday, March 10, 1969

Being that we live so close to the school, we can leave the house five minutes before nine o'clock and still arrive at school on time. We use this extra time in the morning to see Leibishl off on the van. Again, Raizy and I take turns, alternating days, one day Raizy, one day me. It is an easy task compared to those days we would come home every lunch hour to feed him.

In the winter, it is sometimes a test of nerves, however. I dress him in his "seven layers," and when he is finally ready, with his little lunch bag slung around his shoulders, we sit by the window and wait for the van to come. Leibish gets bored, especially when the bus is late, and he starts to take off his hat, then his scarf, and if I still have not noticed, the coat is next. I try not to lose my cool and patiently dress him again.

Once again, we have our noses pressed to the window, looking out for that van. Leibish starts to undress himself again. This time I am getting fed up and I say, "Leibish, not again! Please don't take off your hat, the van will be here soon." It is like talking to the wall. He continues as if I had not said anything. The hat goes on and off his head thirty times. I cannot make him understand to keep it on. Just when I am getting real mad, and Leibish sees me puckering my forehead and pursing my lips into a classical state of a "fit," he toddles over to me and throws his arms (now free of his bag and coat) around me and plants a huge, wet kiss on my cheek. What he can't say in words, he expresses in actions better than the greatest orator. Of course, I am no longer angry; he has done to my anger what the sun does to butter. So once again, I start dressing him while thinking, "Leibish, maybe some day you will learn . . ."

Motzai Shabbos, March 22, 1969

Havdalah has become an event in itself. Leibish goes through the entire routine. By *besamim*, as the jar of herbs gets passed around for everyone to sniff and make the *berachah*, Leibish lets out a long "ahhh" and looks as if he would inhale it all if he could. By *Borei Me'orei Ha'eish* he says "yight" and indicates he wants to be picked up so he could shut the light.

Then he too, rotates his little hands at the conclusion of the *berachah*. As we witness this miracle of Leibish's progress, we all wish each other a *"gut voch,"* our hearts brimming with joy and good cheer. Leibish has us off to another very good week.

Taunting

▼

Today, Mommy came home with yet another little story about Leibish. We are beginning to anticipate these accounts as part of the day. Leibish is the only Down's Syndrome child in the neighborhood, and that makes the whole situation all the more difficult. Very often, people, especially children, tease and make fun of Leibish. Do they think we are deaf or don't care to see our Leibish being harassed? Don't they realize he has a family that loves him and feels hurt when he is hurt?

"Is Down's Syndrome so rare?" I asked Tatty just last week. "How is it that I hardly ever see such children?"

It was *Motzai Shabbos*, and we were home alone, just the two of us, watching Leibish. Lezer was at Pirchei, and Mommy was out with Raizy visiting Etty and her adorable little kids. Whenever Mommy would announce that she was going over to Etty, we would beg, "Please, Mommy, Raizy went last time, Lezer went the other time . . ." Lately, we have worked out a

85

system. There is a chart on our bedroom wall, with our names prominently displayed in large letters. No one gets to go twice in a row (unless the family goes together). We make sure Etty doesn't notice the chart. Who knows? It might go to her head. Enough that she sees our frank adoration of her children, as it is.

We haven't decided yet who is cuter. Is it Chany, the "big grool" (girl), as she calls herself? (She is all of three years old.) Is it Dovidl, a lively two-year-old, who gets into everything and loves to clown around wearing his mother's *tichel* and "fancy shoosies"? Or is it Yoiny, who is certainly the smartest one-year-old around? He has been walking since ten months old and can say quite a few words. You just have to be nearly as smart as him to understand. When he commands from his high chair, "Botty! Cookie!" I come as fast as lightning to execute his orders. What a "tyrant in the high chair"! I guess they are each the cutest in their own fashion.

Tatty brought me back from my musings. "Rochelle, you ask a very good question. The unhappy truth is that there are many children like our dear little Leibishl all over the world, and our community is no exception."

"So where are they?" I asked, more curious than ever.

"In special homes and institutions established for children with various mental problems," he answered.

"But how can you compare being in those institutions, filled with a cold and indifferent staff, to a life at home? Who can take the place of a mother to those children who need love and affection a least as much as normal children, probably much more? And besides, are any of those homes Jewish?"

Tatty sighed. "Unfortunately, no Jewish home of that kind has yet been established."

"But isn't it awful to let these Jewish *neshamalach* eat

treifos and deprive them of a Jewish atmosphere?" I persisted.

"Yes, Rochelle, it is a terrible but real fact. Most parents who find themselves with a retarded child feel they cannot face the hardships that come with raising such children. Furthermore, most people live under the misconceptions that Down's Syndrome is a hereditary condition. They are afraid that if people find out they will not want their children to marry the siblings of this child. If only more people understood that Down's Syndrome is a not a congenital disorder but rather a 'mistake of nature,' so to speak! I add 'so to speak' because you surely know, Rochelle, there are no such things as mistakes. Everything is ordained Above, with good reason."

"Aren't we lucky to have had the good sense to keep Leibish?" I exclaimed.

"You bet!" my father said enthusiastically. "I relish the peace of mind that our decision gave me. Mommy and I are certain that if we would have given up Leibish, Heaven forbid, our consciences would not have let us enjoy a moment's tranquility."

All this went through my mind as I braced myself for this "new little story" my mother had to tell us.

It turned out that Leibish was playing on the corner, near Mommy's shop. Our house is down the block, and Leibish is free to play anywhere within that range. When Mommy noticed a small commotion outside, she was quick to investigate. Outside, she saw a group of boisterous boys. As she came closer, she realized, to her consternation, that they were taunting her little son. How pathetic Leibish looked as he stood defenseless against those callous children. "You have such funny eyes. Ha, ha, ha." They shoved and pushed him in disgust. My mother was furious. She clutched Leibish to her bosom protectively. "Don't listen to those naughty boys," she tried to soothe her little son. Suddenly, Leibish turned to his mother, "They stupid!"

Had they been pelted with stones, the boys would not have been as stunned. Their disgrace was complete. They turned and fled, their heads bowed in shame.

Mommy ended her narration with pride in her voice. "My little Leibish, not yet five years old comprehended that those 'normal' boys were stupid. He is very hurt when kids mock him and does not understand why. He cannot see what makes them be so cruel to him when he is so gentle and loving to others. So the only explanation he can find for this senseless pain they inflict on him is that they are plain *stupid*."

As much as we were proud of him, we hurt even more. How unfortunate that he had to suffer for his handicaps, through no fault of his. We resolved to defend him whenever possible.

Motzai Shabbos, May 17, 1969

Our resolve has already brought action. Lezer, feeling personally responsible for his little brother, decided he has had it with the Blau boys, Tzvi and Moishy, six-year-old twins, who thought teasing Leibish a great sport. *Shabbos* morning during *Krias Hatorah*, Lezer was outside playing with his friends, all the while keeping a watchful eye on Leibish. When he noticed the Blau twins coming out of *shul*, Lezer tensed, ready for battle. As soon as Tzvi, the tougher of the two, advanced towards Leibish, a mischievous grin on his face, Lezer grabbed him and shook him violently.

"Please stop," Tzvi begged. "I didn't do anything."

"Don't you ever bother my brother again! If I ever catch you teasing him, I will hurt you a lot worse."

Having said that, he let go of Tzvi but not without first giving him a strong shove that nearly knocked him to the ground.

That was not the end of it. Tzvi ran crying hysterically into *shul* to find his father. When Mr. Blau beheld his son, he was quick to investigate. When told that it was Lezer who had hurt his little boy, Mr. Blau was furious. He ran out of *shul* and found Lezer holding his Leibish protectively. Without even thinking, Mr. Blau slapped Lezer across the face.

"What right do you have to hit my little *yingele*?" he shouted. "Why don't you pick on someone your own size!"

Lezer was mortified. He had never been slapped before. Ever since he could remember, he had always tried to be especially good. Many times, he felt like joining some good old-fashioned trouble in school or foregoing studying for some tedious test. But then he remembered, "How can I cause my parents heartache, when they have a child like Leibish?" Inevitably, he would stop short and resist his mischievous schemes. He subconsciously felt it his duty to protect his parents from further trouble. Some responsibility to carry around when you are a lively little boy!

Mr. Blau felt terrible. He had not intended to hit Lezer. He was a gentle man who loved children and enjoyed giving out candies on *Shabbos*, provided the children promised to make a loud *berachah* so he could answer *Amen*. He begged Lezer to forgive him and asked Lezer to explain what happened. When Lezer complied, Mr. Blau apologized for his thoughtless boys.

"I must try to impress upon them how painful it is for Leibish when they taunt him," he said. "Just because he does not strike back, does not mean he does not feel any pain. He is capable of hurting as much as any normal child. However, I have some advice for you, Lezer. Inasmuch as I know you mean well and feel responsible for your brother, you must learn to control yourself. Look what happened when I lost control for a moment and hit you. I feel very sorry. All too often you will find yourself angry at other people on account of little Leibishl. But don't stoop to their insensitive behavior. Stand above them with dignity, and you will make them feel worse than through any harsh words or physical beatings."

More weddings

▼

The inevitable has happened. As soon as Shloimy got married, when I prepared to write down everything about it, I could not find my little diary. Ahem, it's not so little. By now it is a five volume affair, held together by a bunch of rubber bands. How I could misplace such a large bundle is beyond me. A full year passed. Raizy was engaged and married, and still no diary in sight.

I had almost given up finding it, having searched everywhere, when Raizy reminded me that I probably must have left it in Etty's house. I once took it there, figuring I would put it in order while the kids slept. The kids didn't sleep, and I had to put it out of the way before little Yoiny decided to try out his artistic talents on it. I managed to hide it so well that when it came to leaving it was nowhere in sight, so I left, thinking I would come back another time to look for it. Soon after that, Shloimy got engaged, and in the excitement, I forgot about my missing diary.

91

Now that I remembered, I became alarmed. What if Etty had thrown it out without realizing it was my "treasured document"? It had been wrapped in an old tattered shopping bag, and it was easy to mistake for garbage. I put on my sweater. It was late September, and there was a winter chill in the air. I ran as fast as the wind. I arrived breathless and knocked frantically at the door. Etty, with her baby perched on her hip, and the others tugging at her dress, opened the door. When she saw my distress, she smiled, "What's the matter now? You saw a ghost or something?" I could never get over Etty's cool manner. Will anything ever shake her? I was too upset to think about Etty's steel nerves.

Before I even stepped into the house, I exclaimed, breathless, "Etty, two years ago I left a bundle of papers here. Have you seen them anywhere?"

Etty burst out laughing. "For two years you didn't realize you were missing anything, and all of a sudden you are frantic at its disappearance?"

"C'mon, Etty, don't torture me," I begged. "It is my diary, which I have been keeping ever since Leibish was born. These last two years I was busy working and 'marrying off' Shloimy and Raizy, and I never found the time for it. Now that I can relax again, with all of you married, *baruch Hashem*, I decided to fill in the past few years' events."

Etty decided she would not torture me this time and reassured me that, yes, she found the bundle while *Pesach* cleaning and had meant to give it to me. Somehow, she kept forgetting about it. It was still sitting on top of her closet, intact.

I mumbled my thanks, grabbed the package and ran home to get on with my job of "recording history." There was much to write about, and I promised myself I would be brief, otherwise

I would get tired and would stop in the middle. Here it goes:

Less than two years ago, when Shloimy had not even hit his twentieth birthday, he got engaged to a girl from Monsey named Rifky Gross. She comes from a very *Chassidishe* family, exactly what Shloimy was looking for. She wanted him to wear a *shtreimel,* and he wanted it, too. They seemed to agree on everything. They both wanted to live in Williamsburg, both planned to send their children to the same schools. They even look alike.

Their wedding was beautiful and very *lebedik.* The *kallah* comes from a large family, and I must admit the *Chassidim* have a special *lebedikeit.*

Before we had gotten used to the fact that Rifky was a permanent member of our family, she presented us all with another "permanent member." She gave birth to a beautiful little boy.

It was just like her to have the house sparkling clean, and as she went into labor, three days before *Pesach,* she still managed to give her shiny floor yet another polish. By the time she arrived at the hospital, there was just enough time to make it to the delivery table. She found no need for the "breathing methods" everyone has lately discovered. She has her own breathing techniques. Sweep, breathe. Scrub, huff and puff. It worked fine for her, but I think I will do it the new way.

In no time, she was on the phone, calling about this "very handsome young man" she had heard about while still in the hospital. Her roommate at the hospital had been talking with her mother about her new neighbors. The Schwartz family had just moved next door to her roommate's mother, and they had a son of marriageable age. The mother clucked her tongue about what a catch this Mordechai Schwartz was. Rifky had heard enough. She immediately thought of Raizy, her gorgeous sister-in-law, and embarked on her new mission. Rifky has already plunged into our family affairs with the same zest she goes about all her various responsibilities.

At Raizy's engagement, the *rav* of Mordechai's *shul* was invited to speak. As he approached the podium and began to speak, all the guests fell silent and prepared to listen to his words of wisdom. The *rav* was known for his charisma and for his speaking prowess. He had a dramatic way of expressing himself, flailing his hands as if to make his point clearer.

Leibish, who was seven years old, was also listening intently and watching the *rav* with interest. Just as the *rav* was coming to a particularly sensitive subject and was accelerating his hand gestures, Leibish called out in a loud, distinct voice, "Lezer, *rav* imitate you!"

Everyone burst out laughing, but none more than my family, who knew exactly what Leibish had meant. You see, Lezer, who learned in that *rav's bais midrash*, was always fascinated by his way of speaking. He loved and respected the *rav*, who was a big *talmid chacham*. My parents would have a great time listening and watching how, at the *Shabbos* table, he would repeat a *Dvar Torah* he heard from the *rav*, delivering it with all the gestures and articulations. When Leibish watched the *rav* now, he could not get over how he could imitate Lezer so well. He was so astounded at this "magic" that he could no longer contain himself and just had to let Lezer know.

There were times when we weren't sure if Leibish said something funny on purpose or unintentionally. But there were times when no matter what his intent was, he made us all laugh.

He was always thrilled that he had brought happiness to all around him, and he would laugh along more heartily than anyone. He knew what it felt like when people became cross with him when he had not meant to get them angry. Sometimes his presence was all that was needed to arouse their displeasure. So if he made people laugh (to him laughter means happiness), no matter if he meant to or not, it was always a welcome surprise. Now, that he got such a large crowd to be "happy" with him, he was the proudest little boy around.

With Raizy married, I am the only girl left in the house. It feels kind of funny. Despite all our fighting and squabbling, we are very close sisters. Mordechai is a great guy; Raizy is truly lucky to have "found" him. There is one thing that I still have to work on myself—to forgive him for taking my sister away. But I am happy for my sister, as they seem to be thrilled about each other and are having the time of their lives. They are planning a trip to Eretz Yisrael. Believe it or not, Raizy has never been to Eretz Yisrael. (Nor have I, for that matter. Do you hear me, my future husband, wherever you are?)

No one is as happy as my mother. There is this thing about *chazakah* (when something happens or is done at least three times in a row, it establishes precedent and promises to happen again.) Now that three of her children are married, she can breathe easier. The worry about having problems with our *shidduchim* weighed heavily on her mind. Every time a match was suggested, and when both sides agreed to meet, Mommy would fret, "What if they decide Leibish is reason enough to go back on the *shidduch*?" As date followed date and when Etty, Shloimy and finally Raizy would come closer to the engagement, she would get increasingly agitated. Only when the plate was broken, and happy *mazel tovs* were exchanged by the two families, did Mommy finally relax. At a time when mothers become nervous and tense as they realize what a giant step their child has just taken and what enormous tasks lay before them, Mommy would become calm and collected. Her child was engaged to a wonderful person despite her having kept Leibish home, not having "hidden him in a closet."

She was aware that everyone knew that they had a retarded child. She would not be surprised if in a way it was an asset. She knew from people's comments that many admired how her family treated and accepted Leibish into the family. Yet, she also knew that there were still plenty of ignorant people around who thought Down's Syndrome to be hereditary, and even those that did know it was not, did not want the "apple of their eye" to get involved with a "mental case." This did not bother her too much. Obviously, the people that counted did not care. On the contrary, they were happy that their child was marrying into a family which had their priorities straight and which had learned to deal with life's obstacles with pride and dignity. The rest of them—let them cling to their naivete. "Ignorance is bliss," some say. To my mother, ignorance is a poison that eats its way into society like a worm wriggles itself into a fruit, until the fruit rots away and disintegrates.

December, 1972

Mommy is getting impatient with me. I have seen some, heard about others and refused them all. They were "all right," they would make great husbands, wonderful sons-in-law and terrific brothers-in-law. But for some other family. I still needed to meet the one that would make something click inside me, someone I would feel I could not live without. I knew I was being romantic and perhaps unrealistic. I just had to look around me and see all those girls who had their heads in the clouds and their imaginations out of control; their elusive "Prince Charming" had yet to materialize. They waited, the years passing by, and their looks wilting like flowers under the hot sun. Younger siblings and the neighbors' daughters, for whom they had baby-sat, were all getting married and having children, while these poor romantics were still lingering on, always hoping, always praying. How many times has Etty told us about all her classmates who were still "looking"? They knew all the "available" lists by heart. If you were to call one of them, say Chany, the conversation would go something like this.

"Hey, Chany, I've got a great *shidduch* for you. He is not yet thirty-five, merely a child, and what a catch! He is a very steady sort of guy. Can you imagine, he has been working at the same place for seventeen years! Now that's what I call steadfast. So what if his job is to unpack boxes at a warehouse? It is not what you do but how you do it. You say you have one little question to ask, so shoot. What? His name? Sure. It's Isaac Kaufer."

Chany sighs. "Oh, him? He was my number forty-three. He was from my more recent ones. I doubt five years have gone by since I met him."

Furthermore, I knew that there were those girls who were willing to compromise. I even know someone who settled for a *bachur* with half a nose, and someone who settled for a midget who stood at five feet when he wore his double-soled, orthopedic shoes. They were all happily married. It reminds me of the couple who were so well matched, I bet they were born for each other. He stuttered and was blind, she was deaf and, *lo aleinu*, very unpretty. (Mommy says you must not call a Jewish girl ugly, and since there might be a slight chance that this story is true, and that the girl was Jewish, I must take extra precautions). It did not matter that he stuttered—she could not hear anyway, and as far as she was concerned, his sign language was impeccable. Nor were her looks a problem—he could not see, and in his mind, she was the most beautiful woman in the world.

Jokes aside, it came to a point when Mommy said, "You better catch the boat, or you will miss it."

"But Mommy, I am only nineteen," I countered.

"Now you are nineteen, a flower in full bloom. At twenty you are older, at twenty-one you are older, and at twenty-two you are really older. At that point, you are like a machine which starts depreciating steadily."

Sunday, June 10, 1973

One evening, Tatty came home in a jolly mood. Mr. Simon, his assistant at the restaurant, had mentioned an interesting prospect. The name was Henoch Perkovsky, a *bachur* with an excellent reputation.

The following Tuesday, we met. That Thursday, we met again. And that *Motzai Shabbos* we met again. It was all for form's sake. We knew it was us two forever right from the minute Henoch walked through the door.

So what if our backgrounds were different? How different?

As different as can be—he is Polish, I am Hungarian! Can you imagine two people from such opposite "cultures" actually forming a union? How would the *cholent* look? Would I put beans on one side of the pot, potatoes on the other? Would stuffed cabbage be "*holopches*" or "*toltod kaposto*"? The way we felt about each other, we knew that somehow we would manage.

With a little tuck here and there (I was at an all time low, I weighed one hundred eighteen pounds! To me that is like being suspended in complete weightlessness), Mommy fitted Raizy's wedding gown that she had sewn till it looked as if it was made for me rather than Raizy. We ran through Boro Park as if there were "going out of business" signs in all the store windows. Mommy, as always, believed in "don't do tomorrow what you can do today."

There were still six weeks left to my wedding when I found myself having nothing more to do. So, I concentrated on learning more about becoming a *balabusta*. I knew that once I start my family, all my shorthand, legal language (I am a legal secretary) and secretarial expertise would do little good when it came to putting up a delicious goulash, or when I would want to bake for a *simchah*. I would have to learn the rudiments of baking well enough so that the next day there would be at least ten phone calls with, "Oh, Rochelle, can you please give me the recipe for that out-of-this-world *dobosh-torto!*"

As much as I felt clear-headed at the wedding, wondering all the while how my friends could have claimed that "they don't remember a thing from their own weddings," I see now, as I try to recall all those wonderful details, that I, too, don't remember a thing. But I do remember two things. One of which the dentist rudely reminded the two of us—Henoch and me. When the bill in the amount of two hundred and fifty dollars arrived unannounced in the mail, I recalled immediately how we had waited for the *chasan's* entourage to arrive at the hall. Always very punctual, Henoch was a full hour late for the wedding. None of the guests noticed, since they (the *chasan* and family) still arrived with plenty of time for the reception. But they did not have time for the before-the-*chupah* pictures. I did notice. And as I posed for the before-the-*chupah* pictures, smiling all the while, my heart felt heavy with worry. This was not like my *yekishe chasan*. I sure hoped everything was all right.

As it turned out, everything was all right. There was a minor accident on the way to the hall. The car was smashed, and so was Henoch's front tooth. An emergency appointment at the dentist was hastily arranged, and with little ado, he had filled in the gap so that Henoch was "as good as new." The dentist went through this little operation with great magnanimity, reminding Henoch at every drill and slurp-slurp (of that ominous tube they stick into your mouth deep enough to test your gag reflex) that he was doing him a great favor. The favor turned out to be accompanied by a hefty price, but what was that between friends?

With his teeth aligned once again, Henoch arrived at the hall. He looked none the worse the wear, and he settled into his head-table seat as if he sat there every day. Of course, I did not see all this at the wedding. I was busy sitting on my throne, accepting the hundreds of *mazel tovs* which I was sure I would remember forever, but of which I did not even recall a single one as early as the next day.

No wonder there are pictures and movies at a wedding. I used to complain about the way photographers have taken over the weddings. It is no longer the *baalei simchah* who decide when to do what. Their opinions take a back seat to the ever-important pictures. Posing for them has become as important as the *chupah* itself. I know of a couple whose wedding pictures were destroyed by a fire, and who went through an entire rerun of their wedding for a photo retake! The wife was at the early stages of her second pregnancy, but with the help of a celebrated seamstress, and with a mere few hundred dollars, had her wedding gown resewn to fit her now more "matronly" figure. (This story might be exaggerated, but only by a few inches.)

There is one picture which I feel is worth all the money in the world. I would not go so far as to claim that I would rerun the wedding for it, *chas veshalom*, but I sure am glad there was a way to capture it, so that I could look back and smile, even on a cloudy day when I feel gloomy and down. After the meal, when the dancing was in full swing, and Henoch was sitting in the center of a large circle of his dancing friends and family members, little Leibishl (eight years old) sat himself into the *chasan's* lap, grinning from ear to ear. Henoch hugged him tightly, and for the next half hour, Henoch was swinging Leibish on his lap to the beat of the music. It was hard to tell who felt happier in the other's company. The dancing proceeded with increasing gusto and with new momentum. This child, whom some would have thought best to place in a home, or to at least hide in a closet, was being as exposed to everyone as possible. No, I'm wrong. He wasn't merely exposed, he was celebrated with pride and with glory. This little incident was to the wedding, what the frosting is to a cake. The perfect topping!

Closet Child

Yesterday was our cousin Suri's wedding. It took place in Williamsburg. Although it was not an unusual event, having numerous cousins on both sides of my family, it was still exciting. It was a break from the daily routine, a chance to get away from my little one. Leibish, being ten years old, was excited about all the music he would hear. Live music! What a treat. Sometimes, I have a feeling that music is the center around which his whole life revolves. His room is filled with music paraphernalia, and I am convinced that he owns every Jewish record and tape that was ever sold. With his photographic memory, he remembers who sings on every tape, and in what order the songs follow. No one is allowed to touch his tapes, and lending them out is not his greatest pleasure. He'd rather give you the shirt off his back! On the rare occasion he lends you a tape, he hovers over you till you give up and return it to him.

Realizing this great love for music, Tatty makes sure that his

102

tape recorders and record players are always in working order. This is no small feat. Leibish loves to tinker with his "machinery" and to tape from one to another. Best of all, he loves to tape his own recordings. Unaware of his heavy speech, he thinks his singing extraordinary. Alone in his closed room, he sings at the top of his voice, into a microphone, no less. One can imagine the racket this creates. But no one minds. The family realizes that this is Leibish's only outlet.

Aside from the hours he spends at school, Leibish's social life is almost non-existent. If it were up to him, he probably would be bringing home plenty of friends. He is very popular at school; his cheerfulness and good humor are infectious. Being high functioning with a quick wit, the staff, too, cannot help but adore him. However, Mommy feels that one such child in the house is as much as she can handle. She feels that if Leibish would start bringing home such children, who at times can become very disruptive, it would affect the house unfavorably and cause needless tension and resentment. In addition, she feels it is better for Leibish to spend at least part of the day in a normal environment.

When we arrived at the hall, most of the guests were already there. The music was blaring (when will they learn that the music doesn't have to be as loud as the Liberty Bell?), and the festivities were well under way. As soon as Leibish beheld the band, he rushed over and stood there fascinated. This was pure bliss!

As I stood next to him enjoying his pleasure, I noticed a middle-aged woman observing him intently. A familiar sensation engulfed me. "There we go again," I said to myself bitterly. "Just when I was beginning to have a good time, someone will again upset me on account of Leibish." I faced her defensively.

She introduced herself as Mrs. Schwartz. "You wouldn't mind if we had a little chat in the next room where it is a little quieter?"

"Not at all," I answered. I was relieved at the friendliness in her voice.

When we entered the next room, which was really a storage chamber, her emotions took hold of her, and she burst into tears. I felt very uncomfortable and waited patiently for her to compose herself. Finally, the woman poured out her story.

"Thirteen years ago I, too, gave birth to a child like your brother. My disappointment was great. Having had only one other child, a daughter, I had so much hoped it would be a little *kaddishel*, a son who would grow up to be a *talmid chacham* and give me joy in my old age. I was already close to forty, an age which I knew carried its risks when it came to childbearing. At *lecht tzinden*, I prayed fervently for a healthy child and a smooth delivery. I used to smile when my friends asked me, 'Leichu, tell us the truth, will you be disappointed if it is another girl?'

"'Of course not,' I replied firmly. 'So long as it is sound in body and spirit, I will feel myself the luckiest woman on earth.'"

Having a child of my own, I knew exactly how she felt.

Mrs. Schwartz sighed. "When I realized that my dreams had not come true, that my child was not all I had hoped for, I was devastated. I went into a deep depression, from which I never fully recovered. My friends urged me to join them at the many tea parties and other functions, but I refused. Worst of all, I kept my son Yossi locked up in the house. I hold my head down in shame when I confess that Yossi has never ventured outside, nor has he ever seen the light of day. As much as I knew that it was no secret, I couldn't bring myself to expose him to friends' and neighbors' pitying stares.

"Now that I see how happy your brother is, my heart could break with remorse. I realize how wrong I was all these years to deprive my Yossi of so much that nature and society have to offer. I hurt for all the happiness I held back from him. But it is too late now. The damage has been done."

"No, no, you're mistaken," I urged her. "Yossi is still young, and you can make amends. A lot can be undone. You and Yossi can still learn to enjoy life, and in spite of what you feel now, you will have much *nachas* as you observe the progress he makes in his freer environment."

"Young *veibele*, you are so nice. But no, it is too late. Nevertheless, thank you so much for your kindness and understanding."

Having said that, she started walking away, as if she was afraid if she stood there much longer she would see the truth which she obviously was afraid to face.

"Please, let me give you my phone number," I persisted. "Maybe you will change your mind. Feel free to call me any time. I can even come to your house and take Yossi out myself."

"Okay, I see you are a stubborn young woman," she said pleasantly.

I jotted down my number on a little piece of paper and made sure she put it into her purse.

On the way home, I told Henoch about Mrs. Schwartz and that I had left my number with her. We agreed that we would do everything possible to help her.

As the days passed, we waited anxiously for her phone call. All she needed was to call and ask for help, and we would hop over there to help her bring Yossi out into the world, where he belonged.

When I told Mommy about it, she exclaimed emotionally,

"How lucky we are to have overcome our personal humiliation! I count it as a true blessing to have raised Leibish to become such a happy individual. I do hope this Mrs. Schwartz will call. I'm quite sure all of us would be to happy to help her in any way possible."

We waited for the rest of the week, but as the week ended, we realized Mrs. Schwartz was obviously afraid and is trying to procrastinate. We try to reassure ourselves that we must give it some time.

Wednesday, December 18, 1974

Almost two months have passed, and Mrs. Schwartz has still not called. I am convinced that, indeed, Yossi's future is indeed hopeless. What a shame. I have a feeling Mrs. Schwartz was right. The damage has been done. Not only to Yossi, we think sadly, but even more to herself.

How much she has missed! How unfortunate that she has not learned to enjoy her child, and even more, to have been proud of him. How I wish she would have given me the chance to tell her how much Leibish has contributed to all our lives, to our emotional maturity.

I would have told her of the time Mommy lay in the hospital, recovering from a hernia operation. In the next bed lay a girl, drawn and gaunt, her face ashen.

"Tatty, what is the matter with that girl?" I whispered to Tatty. "She looks very sick."

Tatty sighed. "She is a Jewish girl but not *frum*. Her family seems to have forgotten about her. No one comes to visit as she lays here, dying of lung cancer."

"But Tatty, she is so young. I wouldn't put her past sixteen."

I was overwhelmed with pity for this young dying girl. My instincts were to ignore her. How could I face a dying person? I was all of eighteen, and I had never, *baruch Hashem*, had to deal with such a terrible situation.

But then I remembered Leibish. How many times did people ignore him because they could not bring themselves to talk to this "*nebech*"? Worse, they were afraid of him. If I ignore this girl, I am no better than they are. Here she lies, sick and lonely, without anyone to talk to. I must overcome my false pity.

"Hi! How are you?"

I managed a smile, and suddenly, her drawn face was not so drawn anymore. Her pallor was replaced by a faint tinge of pink. She was smiling, and for a moment, I believed she was fine.

"Thank you," she said. "Today is a pretty good day. I coughed less." She paused to cough a dry, hacking cough.

If this was a pretty good day, I wish such "pretty good days" for all my worst enemies. But I could see that I had brought her immeasurable cheer.

"Don't thank me," I almost blurted out, "thank my special brother."

It was Leibish who had helped me overcome my instincts. He, with his innocence and loving nature, had taught me so much and had helped me that day to gladden a poor, lonely soul. For one tiny moment, a young dying girl had smiled.

Because of a child who, according to some, should have been hidden.

But Mrs. Schwartz, that unfortunate mother, has not called. Rather, she has given in to the terrible stereotype that is still holding our society so tenaciously in its grip.

Hide him.

Shun him.

Better he would have never been born.

One little phone call would have been sufficient. Just enough for me to have told her. "Expose him. Accept him. He is the best thing that could have been born."

Thursday, January 16, 1975

Debbie Bash is a ten-year-old girl who is a mongoloid. She is very well behaved, has been trained for years and is friendly and responsive. She has been attending HASC since four years of age and has shown remarkable progress in all areas. She is adored by her mother and gets treated with love and care.

Her story would be uneventful and as close to perfect as can be, considering Debbie's infirmity. But there is a snag—Debbie is going to live in an institution. She doesn't want to, her mother is devastated, yet there is no turning back. A state-run institution for the mentally handicapped has already been contacted and arrangements have been made. Debbie cries her eyes out, her mother's heart is heavy with sorrow but go she must.

This is more or less what Mrs. Bash told Mommy one day when she came into the store. She had not come to buy anything but to speak about her sorrow, and she knew Mommy would understand her better than anyone.

They had met at their children's *Chanukah* play at HASC and had become acquainted. Debbie had performed beautifully;

she said her part loud and clear, and everyone was impressed. She is the same age as Leibish, and in fact, they are friends. Mommy always admired how advanced Debbie was and envisioned her growing up into a poised, self-reliant young woman who would be a true blessing to her parents in her own unique way.

Mr. Bash had another opinion, and he could not be swayed. Ever since Debbie was born, he would have nothing to do with her. He insisted on having her institutionalized directly from the hospital. Debbie showed signs of a slight heart problem and needed some surgery. Mrs. Bash implored her husband that they take her home and nurse her back to health. She promised that as soon as the baby recovered she would place her in a home. She really meant it. She was careful from the start not to get too close to the baby, so that she would not have to suffer when they would be parted.

Try as she might, Mrs. Bash failed to keep a distance from her baby. Little Debbie just grew on her mother. At one month old, she started to smile, a sweet, gentle little smile. She was a good baby. Typical of mongoloid children, she slept most of the time and hardly cried. (Mommy always used to say about Leibish's sleeping through the night at an age when we were up through the night, "Hashem does not hit with two sticks.") In addition, she had none of the eating problems our Leibish was "blessed" with. Even without the necessary stimulation, Debbie started to roll over at six months and played with the rattle, her only toy, soon after.

In the meantime, Mr. Bash kept reminding his wife that it was time to "give her back" (the package's return date was running out). He insisted that he did not want to spend the rest of his life in the company of a "mental retard." He was tired of having her come along everywhere they went. At his age, he countered, when their other children have all been married and had children of their own, he was entitled to some respite. By now, Debbie had completely recovered from her heart problems and was a happy, vivacious child. Mrs. Bash had grown to love her, and her heart ached to keep this "gentle little soul who wanted nothing more than a hug and a smile." She started to consider keeping her at home for good. She tactfully tried to explain to her husband that perhaps it would be a good idea to keep their little daughter. She admitted that she might not "amount to much" (as her husband kept reminding her as someone reminds a patient to take his medicine), but she really did not bother anyone. The government was picking up much of the tab, and she did not see that she would be in anyone's way. Mr. Bash could not be persuaded, and when Debbie was approaching her tenth birthday he presented his wife with an ultimatum, "It's either her or me."

At this part of the story, Mrs. Bash burst into tears. She was beside herself with grief. "At my age, how can I be left alone to fend for myself?" she cried. "I have no income and who would hire a woman approaching her fifty-fifth birthday?"

Mommy waited patiently for her to collect herself. She, too, found it exceedingly hard to keep back the tears that were collecting in her eyes. Who, if not she, could know what it must feel like to be forced to give up her child? Not so long ago, she was offered to be "rid" of her child (the word "rid" was not used, merely implied) and was horrified even at the thought. How much more does it hurt this mother who has no choice in this matter?

"No!" Mommy thought. "Mrs. Bash has a choice. She can still decide to keep her beloved little Debbie and not place her between cold walls without a mother to call her own." In her opinion a child must not be sacrificed for one's husband, no matter what the consequences. Debbie was old enough to understand rejection, and it would break her heart, as well as her mother's. All the work and effort put into her at school and at home would go to waste, as Debbie, her spirits shattered, would suffer a terrible setback.

These thoughts went through Mommy's head as she watched Mrs. Bash, her face hidden between her hands, her body racked by sobs. Her own life flashed through her mind as she thought how lucky she was to have Tatty for her husband. As a girl she had always been treated as second class; rarely was she kissed or told she was loved. For her there was only work, work, work. Her brothers sometimes laughed at her when she pronounced a word wrong in the *siddur*, or when on *Chanukah*, by *Al Hanisim*, she did not know which part to say at *bentching*. It did not occur to anyone that she could not know all this if she was not able to attend Hebrew classes after public school because she had to work at the bakery, work at home, go on errands, every minute of the day.

Years later when she had mastered the *siddur*, and later the *Chumash* and many *halachos* in *Shulchan Aruch*, she would pride herself that everything she learned was through the sweat of her brow. She had taught herself a lot through the years by studying and reviewing on her own every *sefer* that came her way.

Soon came the war with its chaos and pandemonium, and it seemed there was no end to her suffering. Then there came a bright light that dispelled the darkness threatening to engulf her. Chaim Weinfeld entered her life, and she learned how it was to be loved and respected. She knew what it felt to be Number One.

She would go through fire and water for him, she would not give him up for anything in the world. But . . . she would give him up for her child. Nothing would stand between her and her children. A woman can have another husband, but a child has but one mother.

A Special Bar-Mitzvah

▼

Sunday, September 4, 1977

I wish I could write of the splendor and drama that took place
at Leibish's *bar-mitzvah*; how he recited his *pshetel*; how he
read in the Torah and how his friends sang; how *lebedik* it was,
and what a large crowd had come to the dinner, to partake in
their friends' *simchah*.

No, there was no splendor and no drama. In fact there was
not even a dinner. His birthday fell on *Shabbos*, and my parents
made a small simple *kiddush* just for the steady congregants and
for us children. It was summertime, and there were would be
less than two *minyanim*. Mommy declined our offers to bake
and said there would be more than enough. She had baked a few
tortes and ordered some small danishes and egg *kichels*. The
kiddush would be followed by a small sit-down dinner just for
the immediate family.

Well, Mommy came to know what mixed feelings were
about. Everyone that was in Boro Park that *Shabbos* and who

113

knew my family even vaguely came to join in this *simchah*. They felt it their honor to come and partake in this special *bar-mitzvah* and witness a child, for whom the doctors had forecast very gloomy prospects, go up to the *bimah* and be *oleh* as was his right. No doubt my parents felt very honored by the big crowd that had shown up. The problem was, there was not enough cake to go around for all these unexpected guests. I'm sure people didn't even notice; they had not come for the food. But Mommy, her Hungarian blood throbbing within her, was very upset. Not to have enough food at a *simchah* was a nightmare come true.

As Leibish was called up to the Torah, her anxiety about the "cake shortage" vanished instantly. As all the people craned their necks to see this "different" boy actually come up on the *bimah* and say the *Birchos Hatorah*, they were overwhelmed with emotion. I, myself, was overcome when I heard Leibish, his voice clear as a bell, start "*Barchu Es Hashem Hamevorach*." It was as natural to him as it was to say, "Hello, how are you?" His enthusiasm was contagious. As soon as he was through, everyone turned to my parents and wished them a hearty *mazel tov*. It was a *simchah* in the true sense. To us it was the most beautiful performance ever.

Leibish was growing up in many other ways. Ever since Leibish was a little child, he had demonstrated a singular love and compassion for people. Even before he spoke and long before he walked, he would shower everyone with hugs and kisses. Any guest was instantly welcomed by little Leibish, who would run over to the newcomer and plant a big wet kiss on his cheek. We all got a kick out of it, and we thought he was adorable when he did it. As he grew older, his custom did not

change, and no one was spared. Leibish was so sure that they all
loved him and could not even imagine that anyone did not enjoy
his show of affection. And why not? He loved everyone, so of
course, everyone loved him.

My family did not mind it at all. It was a great way for him
to communicate his feelings when he had no other way to let us
know. Strangers, however, did not always receive his wet kisses
quite as he expected. They would look at him with disdain like
he was some little puppy who had just licked their shoes. Leibish
would get very hurt and could not fathom what made them so
displeased with him.

As he grew older, his speech became more fluent, and his
vocabulary grew by leaps and bounds. It was time for him to
learn that there were other ways to express his feelings. As he
approached adolescence, it became a real problem. It is against
our custom for adults to kiss or display affection in any other
physical manner while in public. My parents, therefore, decided
it was time to teach him other, more socially acceptable ways to
behave with strangers and even with his own family. It was not
always easy. When they would admonish him for overdoing his
"kisses," he would look bewildered. How was one to explain
that to love was not permissible? Gradually, my parents got the
message across that while it was all right to kiss and hug some
people on special occasions, like his parents and his relatives, he
would have to learn to greet the other people he loved with a
warm smile and a hearty, "Hi, how are you today?"

So while other boys his age who were nearing their *bar-
mitzvah* were busy studying their *pshetl* and the reading of the
parshah with all its *trop*, Leibish was mastering quite different
but no less important lessons. He did spend some time being
taught how to read the *Birchos Hatorah* with the correct

inflection and without any errors. It was not in vain. He made us all real proud with his performance when he was called up to the Torah. But he was also learning how to be a *"bar-mitzvah bachur"* in many other ways. He was learning how to live as a socially accepted human being who was on his way to adulthood and maturity.

After the *kiddush*, we all crowded around our little brother and told him how proud we were of his *"aliyah"* and how handsome he looked in his new suit and hat. Leibish was beaming, his smile stretched from ear to ear. He shook hands with the men and bowed to us ladies like a true gentleman. Obviously, he had learned. He could now be as gracious and grown up as any other *bar-mitzvah* boy. My parents, without all the fancy psychiatry and other so-called "modern techniques," were able to teach him complex social behavior better than any professional.

Right after *Shabbos*, we all packed our bags and returned to our bungalows. Mommy, too, left for the country with Leibish in tow. This was to be the last summer he would spend with my parents in a bungalow colony. After that, he would attend the HASC camp where he would be occupied daily with various exercises and activities. There he would enjoy himself in the company of his friends and be supervised by a competent and caring staff.

Mommy lost no time teaching Leibish all about being a *bar-mitzvah bachur*. She taught him to perfect putting on his *tefillin* daily for *Shachris* and made sure he *davened* every day without skipping any parts.

Soon came *Tisha b'Av*, and Mommy insisted that he fast a whole day. Leibish did not protest; he was proud to be doing what all the adults did. Mommy explained to him in simple language what *Tisha b'Av* is all about, how we mourn for the *Bais Hamikdash* and how we fast and pray that Hashem would rebuild it. Leibish loves to help, and if by his fasting he could help so many of his people, he was glad to oblige.

The ladies in the colony had another opinion going. The same ladies who years before were offering warnings of, "don't bother to train him before he is at least four; don't push him too far, you'll just be disappointed," were just as "generous" now, many years later with their advice. They warned Mommy, "What do you want from him? He is just a child. It is unfair to make him fast. He doesn't even know what this is all about. He might pass out." Mommy was inflexible and did not yield to their pleas. She would continue to treat him as a normal child, as she did her other children, whenever possible.

Sure enough, the fast was off to a good start. In the evening, he went to *shul* to say the *Kinnos*. (He probably skipped here and there, but I wouldn't be surprised if he wasn't the only one.) In the morning, after *Shachris*, he sat on a low stool beside my mother and listened to her reading from *Tzena Urena*. He might have not understood much; to tell the truth, I have a hard time with some of the topics myself. There is no punctuation, and the vernacular used is an old version of the Yiddish we know today. Nevertheless, Leibish loves to sit next to his mother and listen to the melancholy sound of her voice as she recites the endless sorrow and the plight of our nation which still continues to this day. It gives him a better portrait of what *Tisha b'Av* is about than any lengthy lesson, no matter on which level. Sometimes, the tone of voice and the general atmosphere will convey what no words can.

As the day wore on, Mommy began to feel tired, and like

most of the other people, she went inside to lie down. She called to Leibish, who was on the patio watching a ping-pong game. The poor girls knew that on *Tisha b'Av* one must not learn Torah nor perform any chores. To their dismay, they had no choice but to resort to a game of ping-pong. She reminded him that he should not eat nor drink anything and, at the same time, reassured him that in just a few short hours he would be allowed to eat and drink to his heart's content. She patted his head and told him how proud she was of her "big *bachurl*."

When Mommy was up from her nap, the sun was nearly setting, there were less than two hours left to fast. She lost no time in finding Leibish to check how he was feeling. As much as she tried to show her friends that she thought nothing of letting him fast, after all he was past *bar-mitzvah*, she worried inside for her "little baby." To her he was still a baby, and would always be to some extent. But she knew it would be misplaced mercy to protect him from the adult world and keep him as a permanent child. He was growing up in many aspects, and this would be just another step up the ladder.

She found Leibish relaxing on a beach chair. He looked pretty good, considering he had been through almost twenty-four hours of fasting. As she came closer, she discerned that his lips were not quite as dry as they had been earlier in the day. She started suspecting that he might have had something to eat or drink after all, while she was safely tucked in her bed for her nap.

"Leibish, did you have anything to drink today?" she asked gently.

Leibish had a guilty look on his face, but he quickly recovered. "Oh, no way, don't worry, Mommy. I didn't drink. I just noshed a little water."

My mother did not know whether to laugh or cry. She

decided she would laugh. After all, Leibish demonstrated he understood that he shouldn't have had anything to drink. When he was caught in the act, he became his own lawyer. He quickly lessened the charges from "drink" to just having "noshed" a little.

To my mother, "retarded" didn't mean "unable to do things like normal people." It meant literally "slow." Leibish could learn like normal people, but more slowly. This year he had a little sip of water towards the end of the day, but next year he would forego even the little sip and fast like a real grown-up.

No Empty Nest

▼

Monday, May 1, 1978

These days, whenever I go out on the Avenue, I find myself looking out for this handsome, newly-wed couple who happen to be related to me. I can't believe it. My little brother is married. Mind you, my little brother is not so little. He stands two heads taller than me, just short of six feet. But to me he will always be my little brother, the one whom I *shlepped* all over, loving it when people commented on his blue, blue eyes and his golden curls. How Mommy cried when his hair had to come off at three years old! This was after Tatty's cutting most of his hair at night when Mommy was already in bed, to lessen the shock. When he started school, Mommy would run every lunch time to bring him a sandwich because poor Lezerl didn't like the school lunch. The bread was horribly stale, a full day old, and Lezerl was underweight.

The official *vort* was on a Sunday, but they had been unofficially engaged since the night before. We had to keep quiet about it, something I find very hard to do. We had all been employed in the business of finding out all the pertinent data. We held secret meetings, sent out spies and briefed investigators. Everyone came back with the best information. Her performance in school was excellent, both scholastically and in character. I never met her personally, but I was certain I would be pleasantly surprised. Lezer has very good taste—didn't he pick me as his sister?

At the vort, we came to know our future sister-in-law Chavy, and we liked her instantly. Her parents are wonderful people, and there is a cozy atmosphere in the house. Sitting in the living room around the glass table, Chavy's sister, eleven-year-old Chaya, with her long black hair and great big eyes, glanced into the adjoining dining room and when she spotted Leibish, her eyes met Chavy's, almost imperceptibly.

In that instant, Chavy noticed that I saw their unspoken interchange and turning to me she said pleasantly, "Chaya has a cute little story about Leibish." She looked at Chaya and asked, "You mind if I tell Rochel about your encounter with Leibish a few years back?"

Chaya blushed. "Go right ahead, but don't exaggerate. Before I know it you will say that I fainted and was led away by ambulance."

"Well, all right. I'll just say that you passed out momentarily."

Chaya shrugged her shoulders. There was no winning with her big sister. You could tell she couldn't wait to grow up and get back at all these "grown ups." I guess it's not easy being the youngest in the family. Everyone is always smarter, always has the last word.

"We had just moved into this neighborhood," Chavy began,

"having lived before 'on the other side of the tracks.' (Thus called perhaps because of its proximity to the edge of the Jewish neighborhood.) It was a treat to live near the center of Boro Park, just two minutes from all the stores. Chaya was in third grade at that time and took to going out for pizza every Sunday with her best friend Esther Blima. One Sunday, Chaya came home upset, her face tear-streaked and still hiccuping. Upon our worried inquiries as to what happened to have upset her so, she proceeded to tell us that while she was sitting with her friend at the table enjoying their pizza and soda, in came this little boy, somewhat older than them, grabbed the bow out of her hair and ran out of the store. It was a very frightening experience for a little girl, and she said he looked 'a little different.' She had seen him around in the neighborhood and was always very comfortable around him, since he seemed gentle and friendly. So this caught her by complete surprise, and it distressed her to have him snatch something off her person.

"My mother looked surprised and said, 'I see you have the bow in your hair exactly the way it was this morning. Are you sure this wasn't all a fantasy?'

"Chaya smiled through her tears. 'When he peeked into the store and saw me crying, he came running towards me with the bow and placed it on the table. He didn't say anything, but the look in his eyes told me that he was very sorry.'

"Chaya felt bad that she had gotten so upset," Chavy finished her account. "Your brother had meant it as a joke and had hoped Chaya would enjoy his little prank. He must have been very disappointed about the adverse reaction it got. Who knows how many times he tried to make friends with other children but didn't know how to go about it? He must have had a lot of hurt feelings pent up inside him as a child."

"Lezer knew what he was doing," I thought to myself. Chavy was showing remarkable compassion to her new brother-in-law. We could tell that Leibish liked her. His eyes were shining when he wished her *mazel tov* in that gentlemanly way of his and introduced himself as her new *shvuger* (brother-in-law). She had already found a place in our hearts. To us, being nice to Leibish and understanding of his handicap, was synonymous with being considerate and kind; it was a fool-proof yardstick by which we could measure if someone was really nice. Leibish did the endorsing. If he reacted to these people in kind, if he liked them and was comfortable with them, we knew they must have been genuine. Leibish has an uncanny sense of detecting frauds.

Soon after the engagement, we were all off to the country, dragging sewing machines and many yards of material along with us. I sewed my boys gorgeous velvet overalls while Raizy sewed her girls beautiful, frilly gowns with matching pocketbooks. Since we spent the summer together at a bungalow colony up in Liberty, we kept running back and forth between our bungalows, borrowing pins, asking for advice and, most important of all, displaying our masterpieces to each other, accepting graciously as many compliments as possible.

That summer was much too short, with so much to do. This wasn't going to be just a plain wedding of just another sibling. This was the last wedding in our immediate family, after this would be the grandchildren's turn, very exciting no doubt, but nothing beats marrying off a sister or brother. Mommy was probably the least busy, at least as far as her personal attire was concerned. She had already sewn her dress before the summer began, as she was not one to leave things for the last minute.

What about the special *tichel* she would wear to walk the *kallah* up to the *chuppah*? Well, Mommy had her white lace kerchief which she wore to all our weddings, and which she planned to wear to Lezer's wedding. She was always very sentimental about this piece of cloth. To her, it symbolized the challenges and obstacles she had overcome in order to raise this new generation, and this wedding was to be the culmination.

The great day arrived, and it was even better than expected. The *kallah* looked beautiful in her "Scarlett O'Hara gown," and Lezer was probably the handsomest *chasan* ever. It would be superfluous to elaborate on the wedding itself. Whoever meets me on the street stops to rave about how beautiful and elegant it was. There was an aura of emotionalism and sentimentality in the air.

Ordinarily, when a couple marries off their youngest child, someone shows up with a broom and dances with the mother, as if to symbolize that she was cleaning out the house, figuratively speaking, from her children, preparing it for the "empty nest." In this case, there was no place for a broom, the nest was not emptied, nor would it be in all likelihood.

At the *Shabbos sheva berachos*, Mommy and us three daughters found a quiet moment away from the guests. Mommy lowered her voice almost to a whisper, and with her eyes brimming with tears, she said, "Something very strange happened to me. You know the lace kerchief which I felt so sentimental about and wore to all of your weddings? Well, it disappeared. I rummaged through all my closets and drawers. I looked through all the stuff I brought back from the wedding, including my makeup bag and my change of clothing, but it was nowhere to be found. I feel this is a sign that there is no more need for it. It has done its job."

We remained silent. What were we supposed to tell this woman we loved and for whom we felt such sorrow and pain at that moment? We knew that she did not expect an answer, nor did she want sympathy. At that moment, she was a human being who needed to confide about something very painful, and we were there to listen.

Lost and Found

▼

Wednesday, September 27, 1978

Dear Parents,

    As part of our ongoing Travel Training Program, we are training our students to travel on the New York Public Transit System. The program is supervised by the teachers and by our Vocational Rehabilitation Counselor. In order for your son or daughter to participate in this program, kindly sign permission slip below and return it to the school office promptly. Without the permission slip your child will not be permitted to participate in this program.

Sincerely,
Rabbi Stern
Supervisor, HASC

- -

I, C. Weinfeld, hereby permit my son/daughter to participate in the Travel Training Program of the Hebrew Academy for

Special Children, and absolve the Hebrew Academy of responsibility for any accident that may incur during the Travel Training Program.

_____

Parent's signature

Leibish is embarking on a travel program, and we all share his excitement. Imagine, Leibish will actually be learning to board a train and travel on his own anywhere he wishes. Soon I will be able to ask him for directions and will get lost less from now on, hopefully.

Sunday, October 8, 1978

I am still shaken from yesterday's events. Leibish had disappeared, and we were all petrified. The school had little information, aside that they were aware that his class had left on a special traveling assignment, in which the students would be taught to use public transportation. Soon after leaving, the counselor called them distraught saying that Leibish was nowhere to be seen. The school advised him to continue the assignment and take care of the other children, while the administration would notify the family and police.

When my parents were called with the bad news, they in turn called all of us to ask if we had seen Leibish. They reasoned that perhaps Leibish thought it a good idea to drop in on us on the way to the train station. With his limited judgment, he probably did not consider the repercussions such a little visit could have.

We all hurried over to our parents' house to offer reassurance which we ourselves found difficult to feel. Together, we waited anxiously for word about Leibish's whereabouts. As we sat around the kitchen table, I reminded everyone of a little incident that happened when Leibish was around six years old.

Another disappearance: At *shul* the congregants know one another well, having *davened* together in the same *shul* for many years. They are very understanding of my parents' situation and treat Leibish with kindness and consideration. My parents appreciate this immensely. It makes *davening* with Leibish much easier. Tatty has been taking him to *shul* since he was five years old. This may sound old enough, but considering that Leibish only started to walk a little more that a year earlier, and that Leibish still only spoke in clipped sentences, to us it seemed very young.

After a few months of walking to *shul*, Tatty allowed Leibish to wait for him at the corner of our block. Every *Shabbos* morning, as soon as Leibish would be dressed in his *Shabbos* clothes, he would start in his sing song chant, "Bye bye *shul*, bye bye *shul*," almost like a broken record. Tatty decided to ease his impatience by having him wait at the corner a few minutes earlier.

We all knew that he loved to go to *shul*. It gave us all great satisfaction to see how he enjoyed all the Jewish traditions and the *davening* and singing the *Shabbos tefillos*. On *Simchas Torah*, he was thrilled with all the dancing, and he was welcomed into every circle. We never forgot how that insensitive doctor in the delivery room suggested cold heartedly for my mother to just "give him up and forget him." What did he know of the joy and fulfillment Leibish would give us in the years ahead and, *im yirtzeh Hashem*, in the many years to come?

On a cold winter *Shabbos* morning, Tatty left to *shul* a few minutes after Leibish, expecting to find him at the corner. He figured they would continue to *shul* together, just like they'd been doing every *Shabbos* for the last few weeks.

It had been a long hard week crammed with every test imaginable, and we were exhausted. By "we," I mean Raizy and I. Etty was married, and the boys were, most of the time, in *yeshivah* or *shul*. Raizy and I were the only ones who were generally at home. We snuggled back into our warm covers and were determined to catch up on our week's lack of sleep. We hardly had time to close one eye when there was an urgent knock on the door. We ran to the door so that Mommy should not wake up and beheld a very disturbed man in the person of my father.

"Tatty, what happened?" we asked. "You look terrible."

"Leibish is lost, he was not at the corner. Who knows where he wandered off to? He doesn't cross yet himself, and I am petrified at what could have happened to him."

"We'll get dressed in a flash and help you look for him," we replied.

If Mommy would have witnessed how fast we got into those clothes, she would have been shocked. Usually, we would pull on one sock and read two pages, pull on the other sock and read three pages. But not now. Now we were desperate to be dressed and off on the search. We divided our "search team." Tatty would go to *shul* and look for him on the way, and we girls would go off in opposite directions. We made up, no matter what, to be back in time for the *seudah*.

Our search ended in futility, and we came home dejected and worried. Mommy was already up and wondering where we had gone off to so early. Realizing that she was not at all aware of Leibish's disappearance, we saw no reason to upset her needlessly.

There was a knock on the door, and we dashed to it at once. There stood Tatty, beaming, with little Leibish besides him. Leibish seemed very smug about himself.

"Leibish *shul* m'self!" he proudly announced.

Apparently, he had decided to go off to *shul* by himself. "If Tatty wanted to be late for *davening*," he must have reasoned, "that's all right with me. But he can't expect me to be late, too." (Had he worn a watch and had he known how to tell time he would have observed that it was too early—his father being a real *yeke*!)

We all laughed as we recalled this little story that had such a happy ending, and we encouraged each other that this too would end well and we'd be able to *"fartzeilen in freiden"* (literally translated, "tell it in happiness") as the Yiddish saying goes.

As the morning turned into afternoon, we gradually left for our homes. Our hearts were heavy with worry, but our children were due home from school, and we could not stay any longer. We promised to keep in touch about any new developments.

Rushing home, I met my newly-wed brother and his friendly young wife Chavy. It was always a treat meeting them. They had just come back from Manhattan and seemed very amused with what had transpired between them and Leibish.

As they were waiting for the Manhattan-bound B train, they noticed Leibish standing across the platform. He was intent on something. As they looked in wonderment, they discerned his movements and smiled. He was counting his fingers and kept memorizing some instructions repeatedly to himself.

Chavy shouted across the platform, "Hi, Leibish, where are you going?"

"I got to go somewhere, okay?" he announced in that self-important way of his. What an F.B.I. agent he would make!

His train soon came roaring into view, and Leibish, his head held high and shoulders thrown back, boarded the train. What a big man he was!

Mumbling something about making it to Yankele's bus, I ran to the nearest phone and called my parents. Mommy's "hello" sounded tense and expectant.

"Lezer and Chavy saw Leibish boarding the Coney Island-bound B train a few hours ago. He must have gotten impatient with his teacher's instructions and decided to start off on his own. I bet he will be back any minute," I added reassuringly.

"Hey, I think there is someone at the door, hold on," my mother suddenly exclaimed. Sure enough, I heard Leibish give his casual "hello," oblivious to all the turmoil he had precipitated. Mommy was so excited, hugging and kissing him, she completely forgot I was still on the line. I hung up, delighted about this fortunate ending and rushed home to call everyone. Oh, and of course to Yankele's bus.

Today Mommy called me. She chuckled, "Rabbi Kahn just phoned me. He thought I would like to share Leibish's latest quip. When Leibish came to school in the morning, the teacher bombarded him with, ' Leibish where were you yesterday? You were lost and we couldn't find you. Don't ever do that again!'

" 'What do you mean?' asked Leibish indignantly. 'I didn't do anything. I wasn't lost, *you* were lost!'"

Rabbi Kahn suggested that next time Leibish, instead of the teacher, should take the class.

A Golden Heart

▼

Motzai Shabbos, May 5, 1979

I called Raizy. "Hi! How did it go yesterday at Bais Devora? Did you manage to get Sarale into Morah Shila's class? What about the tuition? Did you explain that you are in a financial bind? Oh, I forgot, you had to deal with Rabbi Katz."

Rabbi Katz is the administrator at Bais Devora. He is a tough man, who chooses to be very difficult, almost mean, at times. What a place for such a man to work in, I sometimes wonder. I guess having to deal with us Boro Park ladies on a daily basis one learns to keep an austere demeanor. So far, I have not had to deal with him personally. My oldest daughter is just a few months old.

"You won't believe it, Rochel," Raizy replied. "Rabbi Katz was extremely patient with me, and he demanded even lower tuition than I paid last year for my Tzirele. As I prepared to leave, he suddenly asked, 'Aren't you wondering why I am so nice to you?'

" 'Well, I certainly appreciate it.'

" 'The truth is, this is all because of your brother Leibish.'

" 'Leibish?' I asked, curious. 'What has he to do with my registering my daughter?'

" 'As you know,' he began, 'I suffer from a bad case of arthritis. Lately, I am finding it increasingly difficult to walk, especially to climb stairs. The other day, I was standing at the foot of a steep staircase, wondering how I would make it up, but too proud to ask anyone for help. People were running up and down the stairs, never once asking me if I needed help. I was trying to muster up the courage to ask someone for help, a very difficult thing for me to do, as you know how stubborn and independent I am. Just then, I saw your brother Leibish staring at me from just a few feet away. I asked, irritated, 'Why are you staring? What's so interesting about a sick, clumsy man? Go somewhere else to stare, you *mechutzaf*!'

"Rabbi Katz expected Leibish to scamper away like all the other kids to whom he spoke in that sullen way. Leibish, however, continued standing there for a few more minutes, and then he slowly and apprehensively approached Rabbi Katz.

" 'Eh Eh, Rab..Rabbi Katz, I want to help you up the stairs.'

" 'I let your brother help me and was very moved by his unassuming kindness. You can't imagine with what gentleness he held my hand and led me patiently up the stairs, one step at a time. How much nobler he is than the average person! Even when someone does a kindness he does it for a compliment. Or when he is on a higher level, he does it to assuage his conscience and to gain another *mitzvah* in his merit—a very lofty purpose, don't get me wrong. Leibish, however, had no personal grounds for his actions. His act was completely unselfish. I believe he possesses a very high *neshamah* and has a heart of gold. He simply could not tolerate my suffering and offered his help while overlooking the humiliation I caused him in the process.'

"So you see, Rochel," Raizy concluded, "we thought we were so high and mighty, and meanwhile Leibish here put us all to shame. I doubt I would have withstood Rabbi Katz's offensive attitude. I probably would have thought to myself, 'Listen here, old sourpuss, I looked to see if I could help you, but instead you suspected me of being a *mechutzaf*. Forget it. I don't care if you stand there all night. Maybe it's time you learned a lesson in courtesy!'"

I agreed with Raizy that I, too, would have come out way behind Leibish.

We have long since learned of Leibish's "golden heart." Ever since Leibish was old enough, he has always held his nieces and nephews with utmost tenderness. Our babies love him and respond to his warmth and gentleness. We feel happy when we see how he enjoys visiting our homes and playing with our children. Never will any child move away when finding himself seated next to him. It gives Leibish much joy to feel so wanted and loved. Not that we sit down to explain to our children why they must be kind to him. They genuinely like him and, like all kids, learn to accept his shortcomings as just part of Leibish. This is him, and they welcome him part and parcel.

Chol Hamoed is incomplete if Leibish does not come along. Of course, we don't get him every day. We each get a turn, while Leibish relishes the fact that we are fighting over him, and Mommy gets to have a little break.

With all the love and joy he gives us, there is always the sad truth that Leibish is home forever, without any hope of marrying and leaving behind him an "Empty Nest." When all my parents' friends can finally enjoy some peace and quiet and go off on vacation at will, mine are always tied down with their child that will never quite fully grow up. There is hardly a *Shabbos* or *Yom Tov* without him (except when HASC, in their infinite wisdom, arranges a *Shabbaton* or a *Simchas Torah* up in the mountains). Even when my parents leave on a trip, he is either with them, or in their thoughts. Mommy told me just the other day that she can never truly have a vacation from him. With him is joy, but at the same time hardship—after all is said and done, Leibish is still basically a child who must be taught and admonished constantly. Away from him, she is worried. She misses him terribly and admits that when she is away from all of us the only one she really misses and worries about is Leibish.

Anyone seeing him on the street thinks to himself, "Oh, poor parents, how they must suffer! How glad they would be if he was not theirs." They would be shocked to hear how my parents enjoy him and love him so. To strangers, Leibish seems a tragedy, and something one could live without, but to us Leibish is a dear human being who arouses in his parents a love and concern far greater and more intense than they ever felt for any of their other children.

Slowly but Surely

▼

Motzai Shabbos, February 2, 1980

Over the years, I have collected quite a few of Leibish's witticisms and *chachmos* and have recorded some. Some of the noteworthy letters and forms that have come my way concerning Leibish, have found their way a step further—into my drawer of the miscellaneous memorablilia. As I skimmed through them and as my mind ticked off some of my mental "record" of the past, the resemblance between Leibish and the other members of my family becomes ever sharper and clearer, despite the typical features of Down's Syndrome. In character, too, Leibish has shown remarkable similarities to the rest of us. My father has a wonderful sense of humor; he can repeat a joke many times and we will always laugh as if it was the first time. Leibish, in his limited capacity, has always displayed a sense of humor, just another sign that he resembles his parents more than just in looks.

At my nephew's *bar-mitzvah*, I decided to tease him and

asked, pretending I was surprised he came, "Leibish, why did you come to the *bar-mitzvah*?"

I expected him to retort indignantly, "What do you mean? I am the uncle!" Instead, he decided to play my game. "I came because of the pictures," he replied.

Lezer was asking Leibish when he would be back from *shul*. Leibish has this thing that he doesn't like to be questioned about his comings and goings. He pretended not to hear, but Lezer didn't give up. He kept asking in a monotone, "*Ven, Leibish, ven*?" ("When, Leibish, when?")

Leibish stayed calm and finally answered, "*Ven?*"

So Lezer repeated, "*Ya, ven?*" ("Yes, when?")

"Dodge Van, that's *ven*!" Leibish replied.

As a young child, whenever we would pass the corner of New Utrecht Avenue at the triple intersection, Leibish would ask, "Why all the lights?" Tatty would point out the cars coming from different directions and how the lights help them know which way they could go. He patiently explained that "those over there are for the cars to go this way, those on the other side are for the cars to go over to that side and those ahead of us are for cars to go there."

Finally, Leibish caught on, and soon it was his turn to explain the complexities of the traffic system. He would begin, "You see the lights over there, it's for the cars to go over there (hands would dramatically be thrust to the right) and those on the other side." We would all burst out laughing as we realized what a great mimic he was. Over the years, it became a family joke; approaching New Utrecht Avenue would invariably remind us of Leibish and his antics.

During my engagement period, Leibish was nine years old and was going through a period of naughtiness. Mommy had a hard time disciplining him. As the wedding approached, Mommy used it as a threat, "If you don't go to sleep on time, you will not go to Rochelle's wedding!" It worked well. Leibish would not miss my wedding for anything in the world. The day after the wedding, my mother couldn't get him to finish his breakfast. (Yes, Leibish is still a very finicky eater, although much better than he used to be.) Leibish looked up to see what his mother had to say in the matter, and sure enough, he noted that she was preparing to reprimand him. He offered this advice, "Now say that I will not go to the *sheva berachos*."

Not everyone is so amused by his sense of humor. At school, Leibish could become quite mischievous from time to time. Although we know he must be reprimanded, between you and me, I was amused. He is not at all like the "professionals" describe them, "Children with Down's Syndrome are gentle and placid," as if they were some puppets in a show.

Mr. Weinstein was obviously quite annoyed with Leibish, that year Leibish "graced" his class. In his comments, he dubbed him the "class clown . . . the class leader." When he takes attendance everyone is supposed to answer, "Present." Leibish decided he would take over, and as the teacher calls out the names, he mutters out loud, "Present post." Although I don't really know what he meant by that, the children were amused, nevertheless, and they all burst out laughing.

I can see Mr. Weinstein's puckered forehead as he wrote these words in his monthly report. "He insists on wheeling Esther Gluck around in middle of class (Esther Gluck is an invalid in Leibish's class who is wheel-chair bound), and he always has a ready excuse why he cannot or will not clean up after lunch." (In my humble opinion, he was afraid he might take away the janitor's job.)

When it came to his academic performance, Mr. Weinstein had to confess that he was at the top of the class. In his words, "Does extraordinarily well on all tests. Volunteers to write the correct answers on the blackboard. Completes assignments without supervision."

Aside from his academic excellence, he has always shown kindness to his peers. In Mr. Weinstein's words, "Is very generous during snack time."

As a sister, I like to think of his positive aspects. I do not condone his mischief, but to me it is all because Leibish is special, and with his above average intelligence (relatively speaking), he probably gets bored while the teacher stalled and explained to the slower students something which he already knew. Besides, being a Weinfeld he couldn't help his spiritedness and sense of humor. For Mr. Weinstein, it would have been much easier if Leibish would sit quietly and unobtrusively in class "like a good little boy," but I, on the other hand, am far happier to hear that he is quick-witted and "on the ball."

    1976
Name: Weinfeld, Leibish
Date of Birth: 7/12/64
Date Tested: 4/5/76
Age: 11-9 months
Tests Administered: Bender Machover
Stanford-Binet L-M   MA 4-8   IQ 48

    Leibish is a thinly-built child of about eleven years whose mien is mongoloid. He has a very light complexion, high cheek bones and small features. He has brown eyes and light brown hair. Leibish was cooperative at the testing session.

(Here there are some technical terms that I cannot decipher.)

Leibish will be able to acquire some meaningful academic subject matter. He can develop the interpersonal skills of sharing, cooperation and respect to the extent that he will be able to adjust to family and community relations. He is a very obedient child and a very controlled child, who rarely acts up. With the proper training, he will be able to make a contribution to his own future economic support.

Leibish's motor abilities and vocabulary have shown remarkable improvement. The strength within his overall functioning lies in his social judgment. He can generally handle himself in self-care matters.

As the school year would end and as we would all come home with our report cards and honor certificates, Leibish too, would come home with "certificates." With all our academic achievements and honorary mentions, I doubt any of them ever made my parents as proud as these test results. Their modest ambitions concerning Leibish were bearing fruit. He was already on his way to becoming a valuable member of society.

I stress modest, as my parents don't wait for miracles and do not keep their heads in the clouds. Their feet are firmly planted in the ground, and they keep their visions of Leibish's future clear and realistic. I know that there are some people with DS (Down's Syndrome) who have far outperformed and have displayed higher IQ's than my brother. But this is not a race between Leibish and others, whether normal or mentally disabled. It is a race between Leibish and himself. I am just as proud when he learns to add and subtract or to *daven* a new part in the *siddur*, as I would be if he had a higher IQ and would be learning algebra.

There is a line in *Mishlei,"Chanoch Lanaar Al pi Darko."* Teach each child according to his abilities. While I am impressed with some children who suffer from the same disabilities and who have attained high levels in academics, I never feel jealous or guilty that we have not done enough with our Leibish, or that we should have pushed him harder. I keep "looking up and down," as Mommy always says. As I look up, I see all that he has become, and as I look down, I realize what he would not have become were it not for my parents and for our joint efforts. How, despite the odds and the pessimism, he has come a long way and will still achieve much more. It might not seem "much more" to someone else, but to me, every little thing he learns and every obstacle he overcomes is magnified many times over by the effort with which it is attained.

Whenever I am in the library, which is quite often, I automatically look to see if there is anything about Down's Syndrome. Unfortunately, there is very little, and the few books I do find are all very technical and not too readable. When I found the book by Nigel Hunt, entitled *The World of Nigel Hunt—The World of a Mongoloid*, I was very excited and I ran home to read it. I find it strange that the same year Leibish was born, Nigel Hunt, then seventeen years old, wrote his own book, describing his life and the adventures he went through from his own, unedited point of view. His father, in the introduction to the book, attests to the fact that he did not revise anything except for eliminating four to five lines which were, in his words, "of a personal nature."

Nigel was an only child who was born to his parents in their low forties. He suffered from Down's Syndrome and was mildly retarded. His father was a school headmaster (the British word for principal). His mother was very ambitious, and even before he could talk she introduced him to the alphabet. By the time he was five, she had effectively taught him to read. After a few years in a school for the mentally disabled, Nigel attended regular classes alongside normal children. At the age of ten, Nigel started to fiddle around with his father's typewriter. All his father had to do was to teach him how to use the shift key, and before long, Nigel could type almost as quickly as his father, while using only two fingers on each hand.

Besides being taught on an intensive one-to-one basis by his tireless parents, Nigel had inherited his father's writing talents and thus reached a level which made history in the field of Down's Syndrome. He could actually proceed to write a book on his own. Besides giving parents of such children new hope, it excited the professionals who were doing research on "mongolism." Never before had they had the chance to view these children from their own viewpoint. They could only assume and speculate. It is no wonder how, even in these modern times, they were still groping in the dark.

It seems everyone at HASC has something nice to say about Leibish. One of his teachers told Mommy how one day she got a haircut. She felt strange coming to school the next day, expecting comments like, "Oh, so you got a haircut? You think you look better in short hair?" Surprisingly, no one noticed her new hairstyle. She felt, "This is how they notice me here, after I've worked with these people all these years?" Sure enough, when she entered Leibish's classroom, who recognized immediately that she got a haircut? You guessed it. Leibish, of course. Not one person from the staff or the students had noticed, not even the secretary with whom she went out for lunch.

"Oh, teacher, you got a haircut?" he exclaimed.

The teacher was delighted, and she asked eagerly, "You like it, Leibish?"

"Yeah, yeah. It's very nice!"

There is a saying, "You can fool all of the people some of the time, you can fool some of the people all of the time, but you can't fool all of the people all of the time." If everyone loves him, if everyone is pleased with his progress, it must be that there is something to it.

The speech therapist wrote in her monthly report, "Leibish is quite friendly. He follows commands well. Linga-musculature appears to be uncommonly strong."

At the *Curriculum Enrichment Program* the teacher was pleased with his art skills. He wrote: "Coloring. Vertical strokes. Staying in line from large shapes to small. Drew all shapes using shape stencils. Can pick out most colors. Able to choose card which did not belong in deck. Colors within lines using unified strokes. He has attained many skills. He cuts well and is even able to cut from a pattern with a bit of assistance."

Sometimes, when I would sit with Leibish for hours on end, trying to explain the homework to him, I used to think, "Forget it, you're wasting your time. It just doesn't seem to go into his head."

"Leibish how much is 12 and 16?" I would say.

He would sit there and try to figure it out, finally answering, "Four." (He had obviously understood the question to mean, "the difference between the two numbers.") The addition symbol was not clear to him. But as I looked through his *Year End Case Review*, I could see that it was not all in vain. It reads as follows:

> *Arithmetic*: Has improved a lot. Can add and subtract very well. Has learned to add by carrying. Knows all coins and values. Knows measurements, time. Is good at simple verbal problems.
>
> *Reading*: Gained proficiency in reading recognition and comprehension. Able to spell phonetically. Understands grammatical usage. Applies given rules to sentence structure and sequences.

Mommy was reading with Leibish in his reader, and when they came to the word "no way" Leibish corrected her, "Mommy, don't say 'no way' so quietly. Say '*No way!*'"

Right before *Pesach* vacation, Mrs. Reiss sent home this letter with Leibish.

> Dear Mr. and Mrs. Weinfeld,
>
> Leibish is a delightful child. His diagnosis shows he has learned to speak slowly and with expression, and to distinguish between important and unimportant parts. He has learned many of the basic concepts as outlined to him and which helped him gain in his reading skills. (No wonder his nieces and nephews love to hear him read to them from their books.)
>
> He speaks clearly with complete sentences; knows direction-position; vocabulary, grammar, etc. The language machine has been a tremendous asset in his learning of word recognition and meaning. (I wonder

what this "language machine" is. It sounds like some kind of magic.)

He is always interested in completing the story he is reading. (No wonder Mr. Weinstein, his last year's reading teacher, had complained that Leibish constantly turns the pages further in the reader to find out what he will eventually learn.)

Mrs. Sputz was Leibish's Hebrew teacher. She is a petite woman who is lively and vivacious. Leibish loved her and didvery well in her class. He identified with her as she is culturally very similar to his own family. It thrilled him to learn how to *daven* from a *siddur*, just like his Tatty does in *shul*. He was eager to learn about *Shabbos* and all the *Yamim Tovim*. Mrs. Sputz wrote in his weekly records.

Student's Name: Weinfeld, Leibish
Teacher: Mrs. Sputz
Subject:Hebrew

10/11/76
Can read in *siddur*; can copy from board; knows all *berachos* on food and when to use them; remembers some *yahadus* after the summer vacation.
11/1/76
Translates one page in reader without help.
11/15/76
Answered the *parshah* questions well.
12/1/76
Transferred to "E" class.
12/15/76
Performed excellently at the *Chanukah* play.

1/1/77
Knew Hebrew words learned this week.
1/15/77
Completed a writing stencil without help.
2/1/77
Learned the concept of *tzedakah, Rosh Chodesh, Yom Tov, Shabbos.*
2/15/77
Knows the *parshah* each week.
3/1/77
Can translate ten pages in *Leshoni.*
4/15/77
Learned to count in Hebrew till ten; learned twenty-five common words, their meaning and translation.

To most people it might not mean much. To a boy in his twelfth year, *Chumash, Mishnayos* and *Gemara,* as well as history and science and many more subjects, are second nature. We don't look at "a boy in his twelfth year." We look at Leibish's twelfth year.

No Friends

▼

Monday, February 1, 1982

I visited my mother today, as I do almost every day. It was Washington's Birthday, and Leibish had a day off from school. I invited him to come over for supper, and he gladly accepted. It was around three o'clock, and as we walked home through Sixteenth Avenue, there were scores of people milling about. The weather was beautiful, a sunny day in February, and everyone was outside enjoying a day off from work. I kept meeting friends and acquaintances, always introducing them to Leibish and trying to include him in conversation whenever possible.

I could sense there was something nagging him, that he was not his usual cheerful self. I tried to ignore it, because sometimes it is hard to guess exactly what he is feeling or thinking about. With all the stereotypes of Down's Syndrome children being forever "docile, gentle and happy," I knew that Leibish had his mood swings just like everyone else. Surely, he fell into the

147

above description most of the time, but not always.

Many a time I have seen him brooding when his nieces and nephews around him were doing and talking about things with which he could not keep up. Some of them were a head shorter than him, and he could still remember when they were born and how he had held them in his hands, and now, not so long after, they have outgrown him suddenly. They were dealing out cards, and he remained an outsider to the game. In his own way, he understood it was not malicious on their part to exclude him. They themselves were in a predicament. If they dealt cards for him, too, then what? He would end up just sitting there, staring into space. True, he could read fluently, but the concept of pairing the cards into sets by order of sequence or similitude was unclear to him. He would not be able to keep up with the game and would feel rotten about it. Leibish had a large sense of self-respect, and no one wanted to hurt it in any way.

So Leibish would busy himself with one of the younger children, either reading a book to the, say, six-year-olds, or picking up one of the babies (there were always some available, *bli ayin hora*) and swinging them gently in his arms. The look on his face said it all. "I know I am different and inferior in some ways, and I don't always like it. I am holding this baby because she doesn't know yet that I am slow and not like the others, and I love her for it."

Had you confronted him at that moment with, "Leibish, does it bother you that you can't keep up with the game at hand?" he would have denied it and pretended he was just fine. I can never get over how closed Leibish can be. But not only when it involves his personal feelings. He will never complain that someone was mean. He will just avoid that person as one avoids the devil. If he would be questioned as to why he does not want to associate with that person, he would just shrug his shoulders and go on to another subject like, "Oh, you got a new scarf?" Had you asked him why he likes someone just then, he would have given you a lengthy reason. He has something in his personality which has him dwell on the positive aspects in life, as opposed to harping on the negative.

Many a time when I found myself in his company, I have had an argument with my sisters, or even occasionally with my husband (shhh, don't tell anyone), about a subject I would not have wanted my parents to know about. Inasmuch as it is a normal phenomenon to argue at times, somehow it would have been an unpleasant feeling to know that my parents would find out about it. Being away from an incident in which people differ, and hearing about it second or third hand, magnifies the episode until, as my father likes to say, "it grows a beard and *payos*." With Leibish around, I am reassured that it is as if the wall was there.

True, the walls have ears and so does Leibish. I do not think that he is an imbecile who is as good as the wall. I know he hears and understands everything that goes on. We have long concluded that his strength lies in his social skills, and communication is one of them. Already at the age of nine, Leibish was assessed by the "Bender Machover" test that social interaction was his forte.

Leibish has a built-in sense of tactfulness, something for which I truly envy him. He will never say anything derogatory about anyone, be it teacher, friend or relative. He does not like to express his preferences for one individual over another, even when pressed to it. It is up to the interrogator to observe his attitude towards that certain individual and conclude from his subtle actions or facial expressions how Leibish feels. And I assure that "interrogator" that he will have a hard time of it. With all my attending various *shiurim* about *lashon hora*, loving one another and being equal to all, I have much to learn from Leibish. I am always aware that he has qualities far above mine, and I respect and admire him immensely. He will never complain that something bothers him, unless it is something concrete, like, "I didn't get a piece of cake."

Well, almost never. This time, as we kept bumping into one friend after another and as he observed the good time I had talking and laughing with them, he could not contain himself any longer. He let out a big sigh and said bitterly, "You have so many friends, and I have no one." I knew that he had plenty of friends at school and at summer camp. What he meant was, "I don't have any friends like you. Normal people who are not in wheel chairs and who don't act silly much of the time. Not one person out there who is the same as the rest of my family and who are respectable members of society counts me in as their friend." He might not have thought it in exactly these words, but to the same effect.

This was something new to me. I have had to deal with people staring and saying insensitive things about Leibish. I had learned to deal with them. Many a time I have stretched my eyes to their capacity, outstaring those morons who saw nothing wrong with gaping at Leibish, their mouths drooling, as if he was a creature from outer space. But now it was Leibish's turn to comment about his difference from others, and I was perplexed. I was at a loss for words which would console my brother who was crying out about his pain and suffering, and I could not deny it.

Just then, along comes Mindy Shafrin. Dear Mindy had been sent there by a special *malach*, of that I am certain. Mindy has something about her that turns sorrow into joy and disillusionment into hope. She always has a nice word and sees everything through a brightly-colored glass, turning dull colors into bright and dazzling hues.

As soon as she noticed us, she broke out in a big smile. "Take a look! It is none other than Rochel. Where have you been all these years?" The fact was that Mindy had just moved to Boro Park from Lakewood, where she had been living since her wedding ten years ago. It was she who had been away for years. It was just like her to break the ice. Just as I thought to myself, "Here comes another one—one more person to prove Leibish right." To my enormous relief, she continued, "And whom do I have the privilege to meet? Leibish Weinfeld, my long lost friend! Do you remember, Leibish, how you used to come with Rochel to my house when you were small, and I would give you ice cream and how you always wanted more?" She lowered her voice so that only Leibish was to hear. "Don't tell anyone, but I only looked forward to Rochel's visits because I knew you would come, too."

Well, if I tell you she made his day, I would be lying. That she made his week or month, I would be understating it. She made his year, his decade, his life. She had proven that he was just imagining it. That he too had friends, and Mindy was just one of many. G-d bless Mindy!

The Subject of Marriage

One of the most painful aspects of raising a Down's Syndrome child is the thought of never being able to marry him or her off. When a child is born, people bless the new parents, "*Mazel tov*, may you have the privilege to raise this child to Torah, *chupah* and *maasim tovim*." With Leibish, I feel that the Torah and *maasim tovim* are most applicable. The Torah is achieved by his performance of many *mitzvos*, including his listening to *Kriyas Hatorah* every single *Shabbos*, Monday and Thursday. *Maasim tovim* come easily—he has a heart of gold and a wonderful disposition. This leaves the *chupah*, an unsurpassable obstacle. (True, there have been rare cases where Down's Syndrome people have been wed and where females with Down's Syndrome have even given birth to children. On one of my research expeditions, I came across a passage stating that there have been "no recorded instances of males with Down's Syndrome having sired children," thus I have inferred

152

that there have been of females. But these exceptions have been negligibly small.)

One of the first things my husband told me when he found out about my brother's condition was about an experience he had in *yeshivah* some years back.

"As a young *bachur*, I learned in an out-of-town *yeshivah* in the Midwest. There were two brothers who came from Israel, where they lived with their grandparents. They were top students, and with their wonderful characters showed promise of a great future ahead of them. Everyone was certain they would grow up to be *gedolei hador*, and their respect for them knew no bounds. They had all the qualifications of *"tzu Gott und tzu leit."* No one ever mentioned anything about their parents; it was as if they never existed. Once, I made a bizarre discovery about these brothers. I noticed a *siddur* belonging to the older brother lying on the *bais midrash* table, with its front flap open. Inside were inscribed the words, "In memory of my parents ___ and ___." I expressed my regrets to my *chavrusa* for this young boy and his brother, who were double orphans, having no one left in this world. My friend's face took on a mysterious expression, and he whispered into my ear, all the while wary of any eavesdroppers.

"'You didn't hear about the two brothers' strange *yichus*?'

"'No, how should I have heard? They don't wear a sign on their jackets proclaiming that they have a strange *yichus*.'

"'Ha, ha, very funny,' he answered. 'I figured you'd know the same way I know.'

"'And how is that?'

"'Well, I was *davening Maariv* a couple of months ago, when the two of them stepped up for *Kaddish Yasom*. Naturally, I was curious which parent they had lost, and when I asked

Moishe Rabinowitz, the know-it-all, he told me a very shocking story.' My friend paused. He loved to turn me on and then wait for the effect it had. The more curious I became, the longer it took for him to continue. 'Well, I see you aren't too interested, so I guess we'll just skip it. Anyway, I've got to go and finish studying for the *Gemara* test.'

"I decided to play his game. 'Okay, Shimon, go right ahead. It really makes no difference to me about their parents. They're gone anyway and no story of yours will bring them back.'

"The trick worked. Shimon could not contain himself. He loved to hear a good story, but he enjoyed telling it even more.

"'You know what, Henoch, I'll tell you about it briefly. I can't stand seeing the curiosity eating at you. What happened was the following: There was a very rich couple living in Los Angeles who had no children. They ran from doctor to doctor and from one *rebbe* to another, always hoping to find the right *shaliach* to intercede on their behalf and help them have the baby they longed for so desperately.

"'Many years passed, but they never gave up. Finally, their wish came true. The wife finally gave birth to a baby boy, and they were ecstatic, their dream had finally materialized. To their dismay, however, they discovered that the child was mentally retarded. Their grief and sorrow were overwhelming; they were inconsolable. When they recovered somewhat from their misfortune, they resolved to keep the child and raise it as best they could. It was not easy, since this was many years ago when there were no schools or facilities for such children.

"'The rich man taught his only child to read and write and even some *Chumash* and *Mishnayos*. In his own way, he came to have some degree of *nachas* from him. The son grew into adulthood, and his parents started considering marriage. They saw this child as their only chance at procreation, and their only hope for establishing future generations. They resolved to find a girl with similar handicaps, who would marry their son, and together they would live in their house. Being wealthy, the parents promised the *shadchanim* that if they found a suitable girl, they would be handsomely compensated and the girl well cared for, for the rest of her life.

"'The *shadchanim* spread their wings far and wide. This opportunity was both interesting and financially rewarding. Before long, one *shadchan* located a poor couple in another city in a far away country who had a girl, who was mentally retarded, and was of compatible age and temperament. A match was struck, and both sets of parents came to an agreement that this would be for the benefit of all concerned. The young couple lived in the house of the young man's parents under close supervision. They were given small and simple tasks to perform in and around the house, with few responsibilities.

"'To the parents' delight, their daughter-in-law gave birth to a healthy son, the pregnancy and childbirth having passed smoothly. The grandparents raised it as their own. Hardly had two more years passed, when another son was born to the couple, and who in turn also joined his brother to be raised and nourished by their doting grandparents.

"'The boys' parents were not forgotten. They were treated with love and affection and were allowed to hold and enjoy their children as much as possible. They were told that everyone belongs to one family and that the grandparents are the parents of all of them. They accepted this, as they knew they could never manage on their own, let alone with babies. And so they lived happily in this arrangement, drawing comfort from each other's companionship and enjoying the extended family.

"'Okay, Henoch. Now that I told you this story, I gotta run.'

"Shimon was off in the blink of an eye, leaving me transfixed in my seat. Wow! This was the most amazing story I had ever heard. Somewhere along the line, I reckoned, the boys' parents must have died. I knew vaguely that mentally disabled people, in general, do not live long. Over the years, I came to learn that this was a fallacy. The reason why many of these children died young was that they were not treated right, being placed in homes where they did not always receive enough attention, did not thrive and slowly languished till they died at an early age. Some had heart conditions and other physical ailments which in those days were not treated properly. But there were many mentally disabled and people with Down's Syndrome in particular, who could live well into their fifties if they were raised in a loving and warm environment.

"I did not delve on the reasons why that special couple passed away at an apparently young age, leaving behind small children. What made a strong impression on me was, the thought of the talent and intelligence those two boys possessed and the Torah that came forth from their lips, all resulting from the marriage of two people who were looked upon as forms of tragedy and affliction when they first entered this world."

This story, which gave me much inspiration, still did not change the sad fact that my brother Leibish in all probability, is going to remain single. While we, his siblings, were getting married, the idea of marriage did not occur to him—he was still very young. At Lezer's wedding he was only fourteen, and the concept did not present itself to him. This winter, however, Etty's oldest daughter got married, and it finally struck Leibish that something was amiss.

It has been some time now that I have presented myself with the thought, "Does Leibish know he is different? Does he know he has a condition shared only by a small section of humanity?" I reminded myself of the book I had read by Nigel Hunt, the British author who had Down's Syndrome. I was so impressed with his use of the English language and that he had himself typewritten his work. With all his intelligence, he makes no mention of his being a "mongoloid." He obviously was never told of his diagnosis and was kept in the dark about why he is different from the people around him.

Recently, a man in the United States who was also affected by Down's Syndrome, wrote his life story, and it was published as part of a source book in conjunction with Jean Edwards, his long time friend who is normal. Unlike Nigel and many other people with Down's Syndrome, David Dawson does know that he has Down's Syndrome and apparently takes it in stride. David wrote his part of the book in longhand, and it is presented thus in the book. I have decided to include the first page, so as to get a feel of what people can actually do despite their limitations.

It begins, "My name is David Leonard Dawson, and I am forty-six years old. I live with my mother in Portland, Oregon. I am a person with Down's Syndrome. When I was born in 1936, Dr. Henricks told my mother it would be best to put me in an institution, but she said "No." My mother says that when we were born (I am a twin, my brother Doug is three minutes younger than I) we were both healthy. I weighed five pounds and fourteen ounces and my brother Doug weighed six pounds and ten ounces.

"When I was two weeks old, Mother did notice some differences. I had smaller ears than Doug."

He goes on to tell how his mother did everything for him to grow up as near to normal as his twin brother. "When Doug turned over, Mommy rolled me over, too." It is very interesting to learn of a woman who, almost fifty years ago, used her mother's intuition to stimulate her son right from the start just like professionals today realize what early intervention and stimulation can generate in these children. Furthermore, Mrs. Dawson, David's mother, obviously chose to tell her son why he was different and why he could not do and accomplish what his twin brother could.

To me, it is always an interesting point that the same people who are different, and supposedly can do less than others, in some ways do more. Where is David's normal brother, who was so much smarter and more advanced? As far as I'm concerned, he was just another person who faded into the mass of humanity. It is David, with his mental handicap and overall retardation, who has left an everlasting memento of his life. He has made a mark and has not faded away like his brother.

Whatever the case is and philosophy aside, Leibish apparently does not know there is something basically wrong with him which keeps him from getting married like other people. I'm sure he feels left out and different many times, but I doubt he can put his finger on anything specific. My parents don't think it will make a difference in any way if Leibish learns that he has a label "Down's Syndrome" attached to him, like the coat he just got.

"Mommy, I want to get married. I am the uncle, and why should my niece get married before me?"

This million dollar question caught my mother off guard. After a few seconds, she composed herself and answered as calmly as she could pretend to be, "A niece can get married before an uncle, because girls marry younger than boys."

"But I want to get married!" Leibish insisted.

Leibish felt that if he insisted he would get his wish, much as he got the French toast every Sunday, even when his mother would claim it was time to stop these "fattening breakfasts." Didn't he notice how his belly was turning to pot?

"Well, Leibish, there are a lot of things you must learn before you can get married."

She proceeded to remind Leibish that he must first master tying his shoe laces, must learn to get dressed in the morning without being prodded every minute to hurry up and many more things that Leibish knew he must improve on.

When the list threatened to get even longer, Leibish interrupted her, "Okay, okay, I heard you already. But what can I do? That's the way I am."

It hurt. It hurt badly to hear these sad words. Obviously, Leibish understood he was different and felt inferior when he realized how his younger nieces and nephews were slowly outgrowing him one by one. My mother hid her emotions and exclaimed, "Oh no, Leibish! That's not the way you are. You are a smart boy, and you can learn a lot."

A big smile spread across his gentle face and he let out a whoop. "You mean it, Mommy? I'm really smart?"

We all smiled. The subject of marriage had skillfully been evaded. At least for the meantime. What's more, Leibish came away feeling thrilled with the fact that there was someone who loved him dearly, who said he was smart, who gave him the courage to go on and conquer new fronts.

Workshop

▼

There was not much deciding involved; there was nothing else to consider. Leibish was finished with formal schooling. HASC had given him all it had and had contributed greatly to his growth and maturation. It was time to move on. The object of finding him work was not financial; it was to offer him a simulated work environment and work experience while being in a controlled setting, under a dedicated staff especially trained in working with handicapped persons.

My parents were well aware of the disadvantages of these so called "workshops." The work is routine and unchallenging. The jobs are so specific that they are not really preparatory to any real jobs out there in the real world. However, they realized that Leibish would learn the basic work ethics, namely, being punctual, taking on responsibility, learning to use basic equipment and how to sort, collate and assemble. Many people attending these workshops graduate to regular, full-time jobs in

160

the normal job market, taking home a regular salary. The jobs are simple and sometimes menial, but considering the conditions and the prognoses these people have gone through, it is a very high rung on the development ladder.

Leibish is proud to go to work every morning. At the end of the week, he comes home with a paycheck which he deposits in his savings account. He shares his plans with us. "I am going to buy Tatty a Buick, not like Mordechai's (Raizy's husband) which is such a jalopy. I will get Tatty a brand new one, with four doors and cushioned seats." We ask him if he has enough money. "Sure," he tells us. "I already deposited many checks in my bank." When we ask how much money he already saved up, he hesitates before he says, "I have plenty."

Leibish does not understand what money is all about. He knows that it is a means of purchasing goods. He understands you can't just go into a store and ask for something without payment, but he has no idea about the value, or for that matter how to figure out how much change he should get back. Mommy claims that the reason is that he has no interest in monetary matters. She points out what a phenomenal memory he has when it comes to people's names and cars. How he remembers which person from which family owns which model car and why he got rid of the old one.

He can stand on a busy street corner and direct traffic better than any trained police officer. (Almost.) He calls out, "Hey, you Chevy Nova, turn left; and you, red Cadillac, stop until I give you the right of way." He would go on directing traffic if it wouldn't be for his concerned sister who feels he is drawing unnecessary attention, to say the least, and who yells, "Leibish, get off the intersection and go home. Mommy is waiting for you with supper." When no one familiar is around, a very jealous policeman comes along and threatens to sue for job trespassing.

When it comes to things that engage his interest, he sometimes shows even greater expertise than people of average intelligence. Whatever the reason is for his inability to master economic issues, we must all deal with the fact that he is not ready for a normal work environment and that the workshop is the ideal solution.

His work day is somewhat shorter than the regular eight-hour shift, which is advantageous since Leibish has somewhat less endurance than most people. Lezer likes to say that Leibish is lazy. I claim that he actually has less stamina and, coupled with his sluggish movements, finds tasks more strenuous than other people would, thus making a full time job very exhausting for him.

After workshop, Leibish helps my brother in his pharmacy. He takes care of some deliveries and makes the daily bank deposits. The other day, Leibish decided he had no patience to wait on the before-closing rush hour line. He pushed ahead of everyone all the way to the front of the line, all the while keeping a straight face, as if he saw nothing wrong in what he was doing. People did not respond very favorably and some grumbled out loud. When an older man admonished him for his bad manners, he turned around and said good-naturedly, "I am allowed to because I am crazy."

My parents' neighbor happened to be in the bank just then, and he related what happened to my father. Needless to say, my father scolded Leibish for forgetting his manners and for saying such a terrible thing about himself when really he was a very nice young man who could do so many things like everyone else. But when Leibish didn't see, Tatty smiled as he told Mommy, "Leibish knows how to take advantage of a situation, even if it takes saying that he is crazy so that he can push himself ahead."

At work, Leibish has a great time. He is surrounded by people of his kind and being above-average functioning, he feels his superiority over his peers and quite naturally assumes leadership. Whenever my father meets Mr. Kahn, the administrator of HASC school/workshop, he gets a rave review about Leibish's performance, and he refers to him as the "boss." No wonder Leibish enjoys going to work; he has great fun there, everyone loves him and he is very popular. It is one place where he counts, where he is not "weird." (No one should think he doesn't know it, by observing the complete contrast of behavior when he is in his own environment and when he is with normal people. One can see at once how much he knows his status in society. Among his own friends he acts more natural and is far more at ease than with strangers who give him the feeling, even when it is not intentional, that he is not like them, that they have something he doesn't. He instinctively tightens up and is far less relaxed.)

It is most fortunate that these workshops were created. In the past, people with mental or physical disabilities had nowhere to turn. There were no jobs available, and the only choice was to let them wander aimlessly with nothing meaningful to fill their lives. Eventually, they would lose their minds completely for lack of stimulation and would be placed in institutions.

I remember when I was little, Mommy bought a new broom for *Pesach*. I chanced to look at the bottom of the broom, right above the bristles, and noticed the inscription. "This article has been produced by the blind." I had been awed at the thought that someone blind, whom I always pictured as just sitting there in a rocking chair and swaying to and fro for lack of anything else to do, could actually have produced this useful product. To me, someone without eyesight had no ability to do anything meaningful in his lifetime. Even with the advent of Braille, when they could finally read and write and learn about the world around them, they couldn't, so I thought, perform any tasks. To think that they could actually produce items to enhance other people's lives was a completely new concept to me. Little did I know then how this same type of workshop, which enabled the blind to be active members of society, would one day accommodate my brother in the same manner, albeit for different reasons.

Whenever I buy a box of nails, a package of colored papers, a set of magic markers, I automatically think of the workshop. I picture Leibish, along with his friends, sitting at a table and carefully collating, sorting and finally packing this same package that I have just bought at Woolworth's. They have a part in my children's and countless other people's everyday life. He has perhaps not become a doctor or a lawyer, has not gotten married nor learned *Shas*, but he has become an asset to society in his own individual way. He has assumed a place in the large puzzle, and without him the jigsaw is incomplete.

One might think, "Well, this is not what I call a purpose in life." True, I could think of more lofty occupations than to sit and pack little jars of, say, buttons. But who is to say that sitting in an office and juggling real estate parcels is so much more elevated? The man who runs around Wall Street, buying and selling junk bonds, what is he accomplishing in life? Has he bettered anyone's lot? Did he in any way improve society's conditions? The man who produces mail advertising, what has he established, besides an ever wary public who knows it is all a fraud and must be very careful lest they, too, be ripped off? At the workshop, the people learn to be very considerate of one another, and to work together within their limited capacity to produce honest and exemplary workmanship. Far more lofty standards than many people can claim.

Brotherly Love

▼

Wednesday, January 2, 1985

My brother Shloimy plays a major role in Leibish's life. He has an unusually kind personality. Even as a youngster he was always there to help out. On *Chol Hamoed* back in those years, over twenty years ago, when he was just past *bar-mitzvah*, he would tour all over New York without my parents being concerned in the least. The subways were safe, the streets not yet the perpetual habitat of hooligans and drug addicts. My parents thought nothing wrong of letting him go by himself almost anywhere he wanted.

He could be found all over the city, visiting places like the court houses, the Statue of Liberty and the Empire State Building with little Lezer perched on his shoulders. He was always ready to take his little brother anywhere he wanted. As he matured, so did his favors and kindness. Whenever any of us needed a ride anywhere or if we ever found ourselves with a "cash flow problem," Shloimy was always there to help. All that was needed was a phone call. No preliminaries were needed, no excuses necessary. If you needed help, Shloimy was always there.

When Leibish came on the scene, Shloimy was in an out-of-town *yeshivah* and was home only on occasion. Even so, he was always ready to babysit, to play with Leibish and to take him out on walks whenever he found himself home. Admittedly, however, in those first years, Raizy and I, who were at home more than the others, played a major role in Leibish's progress. As we all got married and became busy with our families, we came to see how Shloimy was steadily becoming a big part in Leibish's daily life. Leibish was always welcome to visit his home. Rifky, Shloimy's wife, is a great homemaker, and Leibish loves to eat there. In *shul*, Shloimy, knowing how his brother loves nothing more than an *aliyah*, makes sure to buy him one from time to time. He gets much satisfaction when he observes with what enthusiasm and gusto Leibish is *oleh*.

As Leibish finished school and entered the workshop, he became an unofficial employee in Shloimy's pharmacy. He ran deliveries, made the bank deposits and gradually became an indispensable part of his operation. With endless patience, Shloimy would teach him and encourage him with new tasks and responsibilities. Even when Leibish made mistakes, when he mixed up two addresses and switched prescriptions, Shloimy would explain to him how to avoid such mistakes in the future.

By now, as Leibish has been working at the pharmacy after workshop hours for quite a few months, he has become adept at handling many assignments at a time. Last Friday, when we came to say *Gut Shabbos* to my parents, Leibish was hurrying out of the house and would not say where he was off to. He was going "someplace," and that was that. It was no use asking and prying. He was a grown man and did not have to explain every step he took. We respect this need for privacy and leave it at that. Just as he was out the door, Tatty boasted to me how far Leibish has come. That morning, Shloimy had sent him on three different assignments and he had performed *par excellence*. He had no list, no addresses written down, everything was memorized. The addresses he went to were all in opposite directions, and there were some things to pick up, others to deliver. On the way back he still stopped in at the luncheonette to treat his "boss" to his favorite pastry, a cheese danish.

There are other ways Leibish helps out, although indirectly. A couple once came in to order an expensive prescription. They explained that they needed to ask the price because they would be ordering it on a regular basis. A price difference, although small, would amount to a small fortune over an extended period of time. Shloimy quoted a price, and the couple stepped aside and discussed it between themselves. After a short consultation, they went ahead with the order and promised to use his pharmacy on a continuous basis.

"To tell you the truth, Mr. Weinfeld," they added, "your price is a bit higher than the pharmacy on the next block, but we decided to use you anyway. You might not believe us, but your brother is responsible for our decision."

Shloimy was very surprised by all this. First, he had just made a new customer; people who were in need of weekly, very expensive drugs were his best customers. "Someone's gain, is another one's loss." It is an unfortunate phenomenon that my brother's income must be from people who are not well and who must spend so much on their illnesses. My brother is always careful to be especially sympathetic to his customers and keeps in mind that they would rather spend their money elsewhere. He tries to make it as pleasant as possible for all concerned.

Aside from being glad to have just made a new customer, Shloimy was even more curious to hear why they chose him over another, less expensive pharmacist.

"We recently had a wedding in Montreal," the couple related, "and as we were coming off the Montreal-Boro Park bus, we wondered how we would manage with all our luggage. Along comes your brother, and without much ado, he took one suitcase in one hand and a second in the other hand and said, 'Okay, Mister, I'll help you with your packages.' If you have the *zchus* to employ such a brother, we can at least give you some business."

My brother knew how Leibish must have fought with himself when he offered to help this total stranger with his packages. Leibish is by nature somewhat slow and dislikes physical exertion. Even at the workshop, where he does very well and his performance is well above average, he becomes problematic when it comes to packing, unpacking or carrying boxes from one place to another. It takes a lot of persuading and coaxing until he performs these tasks. And yet, here was this couple, whom he never met before and whom he could easily have ignored and continued on his merry way. He was not forced, not even asked to help out with this unpleasant task, which he always tries to avoid. Still, he could not see people suffering through hardship without lending a hand. He looked away from his own discomfort so that he could help others. The other person came before himself. Shloimy was grateful for his brother's selflessness and appreciated his indirect enhancement to his livelihood.

Leibish, too, appreciates his brother in full measure. No one comes before his "big brother Shloimy." Lezer could be in the midst of putting up his *sukkah*, and Leibish is over at his house to help him, but if Shloimy calls up that he needs Leibish to run an errand, Leibish says, "I'm sorry, Lezer, but I gotta go."

"But, Leibish," Lezer begs, "we are almost finished. There are just two more boards left to nail in."

"Sorry, Buster Brown, but Shloimy needs me."

No promises of cream cake and chocolate milk will dissuade him. Lezer somehow finishes the *sukkah*, sweating and toiling, and thinks, "Well, let's face it. Shloimy is his idol, and Leibish has all the right to be loyal to him. He is everything to him, a brother, an employer and a best friend."

Treated as an Adult

▼

Sunday, December 21, 1986

As Leibish grows older, it becomes increasingly more challenging to communicate with him on the appropriate level. When he was small, I spoke to him as to any child. I clapped my hands and "yayed" when he learned a new skill, patted his little blond head when he said please and thank you. When he misbehaved, I showed him how displeased I was, at times pretending to cry so he should really see how his misbehavior grieved me. Even when he was a little older, as old as ten or eleven, I still thought of him as a little boy and saw nothing wrong with speaking to him on a child's level. The fact was, his mental age was still at a five-six year old stage and being much shorter than other kids his age, I had little trouble perceiving him as not much more than half his chronological age.

As he passed *bar-mitzvah* age and grew into adolescence, I could no longer pretend he was a child who would always remain so all his life. True, in some ways I knew he would not

171

grow up the way you and I did, but I had to realize that although his mental age was six, he as a person was not a six-year-old. He will be socially and emotionally very different than a six-year-old. By treating him as younger than his age, he will have no chance to develop any self esteem and dignity.

Yet, I am not fooling myself into thinking that he is now, at the age of twenty-two, no different than any other twenty-two-year-old man. I cannot say to him, "So, Leibish, what do you say to the recent primaries? Do you think Reagan will make it?" But neither can I approach everyone else with this question. There are many people who have very low intelligence and cannot be engaged in anything more intellectual than, "Isn't this cake delicious?" or "Isn't it a beautiful day?" That does not mean that we must speak to them as little children. It would be most inappropriate to ask them, "Mrs. Wolf, were you a good little wife today?" Or, "Mr. Shwebel, how many times must I tell you to wash around your mouth?"

When I do see Leibish with a "ring around his mouth," I don't have to announce in front of everyone that he better wash his face or else. It was all right when he was younger. But now that he is an adult, I must always keep in mind his "emotional" and "social" feelings as well as his chronological age, and act accordingly. At times, I find it necessary to remind him to wipe his nose. It seems to me he does not feel when his nose is full, and sometimes it can become very unpleasant to look at him. My instinct is to admonish him with, "Hey, Leibish, you look horrible. Go get a tissue and wipe your nose this minute!" It might be effective and will do the trick this time. But it will do irreparable damage. It will prove to him that he is nothing more than a little child, and he will act accordingly. I can accomplish much more for the moment as well as for the future, when I pull him aside gently and whisper to him, "Leibish, do me a favor and get a tissue." He can thus keep his dignity and will gladly comply.

Nobody wants to look messy and unkempt, and Leibish is no exception. On the contrary, I can't think of anyone who loves to look good as much as he does. He treasures a new garment and will take very good care of it. Mommy always boasts of how neat and clean he is. He takes infinite care at mealtimes not to soil his clothes. On *Shabbos* and *Yom Tov*, as well as at *simchos*, Leibish is as well dressed as anyone around him. He walks with a dignified step and looks trim and neat in his dark, tailored suit.

We are all relieved that he has not put on excess weight over the years. We are aware that obesity is a common problem of persons with Down's Syndrome. They tend to be less active than most people and do not burn their food to the same extent. Also, they have few interests and, therefore, take great pleasure in their meals. And finally, as these children grow up and the parents find it increasingly hard to teach them new skills and habits, they get frustrated and bribe them with sweets. They might feel guilty when they are impatient and will compensate by giving them a *nosh* to pacify them. When they see how their child is being excluded by the children on the block and ends up watching forlornly from the sidelines, they hurt for their child and will offer it a special treat to counteract the child's disappointment.

Mommy is very health conscious and limits the sweets to a minimum. Leibish knows that the lollies and chocolates my parents keep in a special drawer are reserved for the grandchildren. They explain to him that he is not a child anymore and must watch that he remain slim, so he could continue to look as handsome as he does. When he insists on something fattening,

Mommy reminds him of the new suit he just got for *Yom Tov*, and if he overindulges himself it will not fit him. Very sensible reasoning, in my opinion. Not any different from how she would warn her own dear husband, or any of us for that matter.

Therein lies the key. Not any different from how she would warn any of us. They have always treated Leibish the same as the rest of us. When he displeased them, they punished him, and when he behaved they rewarded him, always in the same manner as if he would be just a regular child. They felt that being too lenient and overprotective because he "was, *nebech*, born like that" was the wrong approach. It might seem harsh to an outsider when they see how strict my parents are sometimes, but what better proof that they know what they're doing than Leibish himself?

People are always expressing their wonder over the tremendous job my parents have done with Leibish. They are amazed how, at a time when keeping such children was so rare and when there was so little information on raising them, my parents have shown such success. They observe his impeccable manners, how he gets called up for an *aliyah* or for *gelilah* at *shul* and performs as well as any other member. Lately, he had taken to treating the others to various *kibbudim*. It gives him infinite pleasure to buy an *aliyah* for a brother or another *shul* member who is always nice to him. Anything he can do to prove himself a "man among men" makes his day.

Tatty is always there to inspire and encourage him in his manly endeavors. It makes my heart burst with pride when, on *Purim*, I see how my father accompanies Leibish on his *mishloach manos* trips. Leibish carries the baskets, laden with cakes and sweets, to all the neighbors and relatives. My father always prepares something original for him to wear. Nothing crazy or absurd. Just a little funny hat or a little mask. Enough to make Leibish feel an important part of the *Purim* scene. Everyone welcomes him with a big smile—it comes easy. Leibish hands the *mishloach manos* with such a flourish, and announces "Happy *Purim*" with such zeal, that everyone breaks out in a big grin and wishes him and my father a very happy *Purim*, indeed.

Leibish shows remarkable dignity at the family *simchos*. (He is always invited personally. He will not settle for anything less than his own personalized invitation. He feels he is his own man and being counted as just "Mr. & Mrs. Weinfeld & Family" is not enough.) At the close weddings, when he is called up to dance with the *kallah*, he hands the money to the *badchan* with much grace and proceeds to take the other end of the *gartel*. He sways gently sideways a couple of times and then joins the circle of men in their dancing. I can see some of the guests from the "other side," who don't know him yet, looking on a little uncomfortably, perhaps afraid he might act silly and inappropriate. They are soon relieved, and very pleasantly surprised at how proper and correct he has conducted himself throughout the performance.

We who know Leibish are not at all surprised. We may know that he comes up short in some things, but when it comes to being a *mensch*, he is always ahead.

A Day at Camp HASC

▼

Thursday, August 6, 1987

Visiting day at Camp HASC is a sacred day. It must not be missed for any reason. Nothing can be more important than coming to Leibish's camp and showing him that we remembered he was there and we have come to see him because we missed him so.

All of us gather at the camp, choosing the largest, most majestic tree for our "camp out," so we could enjoy as much shade as possible from the hot July sun. It is probably Leibish's best day of the summer, or so I like to think. We all bring along some goodies, some cans of soda for Leibish. It is always some time around his birthday, so it turns out to be a sort of birthday party. Even when one of us is right after a baby, the husband and the other children make it their business to come. The camp has beautiful large grounds with ample trees to provide the many visiting families with shade.

Our children look forward to "visiting day at HASC." Our

176

albums are filled with pictures of Leibish, flanked by a large, loving family with everyone smiling and looking real happy. The nieces and nephews have scaled many trees and have raced across the grounds countless times. They seem to be very comfortable around the campers. They don't seem to suffer any uneasiness when they observe the various "special" children, some of them severely handicapped, both mentally and physically. To me, it is a very emotional experience. On the one hand, I am happy to see my brother having the time of his life and hearing his counselors praise him in all ways. On the other hand, now that I have children of my own, I hurt for all those parents out there who have carried their children for nine long months, hoping, wishing and "expecting" in the true sense of the word, a normal and healthy child. I could feel their despair and their pain when they come to visit with their child, and once again come face to face with their grief. Some of them hardly recognize their parents, others are bewildered why they must stay while their parents and siblings leave.

Last year, one little boy carried on so that it tore at my heart. The poor boy, a child of around five or six, affected with Down's Syndrome, was hysterical. He could not speak yet, but he kept pulling at his mother's dress and would not let go. There was no use explaining to him, because he had a hearing problem (DS children are very susceptible to ear infections, due to their small ear canal which collects fluid more easily than those of other children) and was deaf and mute. His parents remained stoic; their other nine children were there, and they had to show them that all was well. They gently pulled him away and with hugs and kisses handed him over to his counselor.

As I looked around this past summer, I found myself greeting many people. Over the years, I had gotten to know quite a few of the campers and their families. Susan, to our right, was sitting by herself, softly chuckling while clasping to her bosom a little rag doll in one hand and a package of goodies in the other. She was around twelve years old. She was moderately retarded and walked with crutches. She lived far away, and only her aunt who resides in Queens could make it up here. She had given her niece the doll and the goodies, and Susan appreciated it, expressing her happiness in her simple way.

Yoiny Reich was sitting with his family at the next table. Joy was written all over his face. And why not? His loving parents were there to visit him along with Shimon, two years younger than him, and Tzirel, who at six was the baby of the family.

I had met Mrs. Reich two summers before in the Camp HASC lobby, while we waited for our children to buy themselves some drinks at the canteen. She was a friendly sort, and before long, we were discussing her Yoiny and my brother Leibish. She was just a few years older than me, but the years and her experiences made her many years wiser. She claimed, although I might find it hard to believe, that she used to be very quiet and reserved as a girl. Even after her wedding, she was still very shy, almost timid. Having Yoiny, who was born with Down's Syndrome, changed everything.

She, like Mommy, first refused to believe that her baby was indeed mongoloid. He was her first child (she was just short of twenty), and she had no other children to compare him to. If he slept a lot, well, many children need a lot of sleep. If that first smile took long to appear, some of her friends who had also given birth recently claimed that their babies were also slow with certain things. But as the months passed by, she began to realize that he was different in so many ways that it was time to face up to it. Her child was not normal, and she would have to muster her courage and come out of her shell. She would have to shed her cloak of reserve and become more bold in her search for help.

Mr. Reich, who had grown up in a sheltered environment all his life, was not familiar with such children, surely not this close to home. He did not stand in the way of bringing Yoiny home, he merely kept away. Mrs. Reich hoped that in time he would warm up and learn to love his firstborn. Yoiny was growing up happily and making steady gains.

Two years after his arrival, another little son was born to them. Before long, as soon as Shimon learned to speak, his first sentence was, "Shimon, too." As little as he was, not yet two, he began to realize that his mother's life revolved around Yoiny. She was forever taking him to speech therapists and special classes. It became a real problem as Mrs. Reich observed Shimon becoming ever more resentful of his older brother. Later, when Shimon was five and Yoiny seven, he was even more vocal about his resentment. His mother would ask him to keep an eye on Yoiny when they played outside on the sidewalk so he should not run into the street. He complained, "If I have to watch Yoiny then I'd rather stay indoors." Finally, she voiced her concern to the social worker at HASC, and he advised her to try to include Shimon in as many activities as she could. Even at the speech therapist, she should ask if Shimon could be given some exercises so that he should not feel so left out.

There was another problem to deal with. Mr. Reich was still staying away from Yoiny, and though he took both boys to *shul* every *Shabbos*, he hardly looked at Yoiny, while he was busy with Shimon, pointing in the *siddur* so that he could keep up with the *baal tefillah*. One *Shabbos* when Yoiny was around seven, Mr. Reich overheard this conversation in *shul*, which was to change his attitude to Yoiny forever.

Mr. Weiss, another congregant, approached Yoiny, who was standing in a corner all by himself. He patted his head and made some conversation with him. Yoiny's eyes lit up. He was a very friendly child and was eager to have someone pay attention to him.

"Yoiny, do you like your mother?" Mr. Weiss asked.

"Yes!" answered Yoiny enthusiastically.

"Do you like your brother?"

"Yes!" A little less enthusiasm, but still with a big smile.

"Do you like your father?"

"No way!"

Mr. Reich heard no more. His eyes misted over, and he felt like two cents. It hit home as no speech from any adult would have. From that day on, Mr. Reich became obsessed with getting his little boy back. He did anything so that Yoiny would never again answer, "No way!"

As I observed the family sitting together, I could see that Mr. Reich had indeed completely won over Yoiny. His son was sitting close to him, leaning his blond head on his shoulder. Yoiny was of medium height with long blond *payos* and a bright expression on his face. Now, at fifteen, Yoiny could learn *Chumash*, and his father had hired a tutor to learn *Mishnayos* with him.

To Mr. Reich, it was very important for his son to know *Mishnayos*. I asked Mrs. Reich how well he understands it all. She was honest and admitted that although he could translate spontaneously many phrases in the *Chumash* and *Mishnayos*, he had a hard time with the abstract meanings and comprehension. One day her husband was testing Yoiny on the translation of the *pasuk "Vayomer Hashem el Moshe."* Yoiny knew it well,

"And Hashem said to Moshe." Mr. Reich decided to go a step further this time, "Who said to Moshe?" Blank. "To whom did he say?" Another blank. But Mr. Reich was not fazed. Yoiny was only fifteen, and with constant tutoring he could still learn a lot more.

I heard little Tzirel tell her mother, "Mommy, you know? I'm so happy that our Yoiny is a little different. Shimon is already *bar-mitzvah*, and he is not interested in my games. He says they're 'babyish.' When it is a rainy *Shabbos*, I would be so bored. None of the neighbors come over to play with me, and it gets lonely all by myself. Yoiny is always there to keep me company. He never complains that he is too big to play with this or that." At this point they passed out of earshot; Mrs. Reich was taking her little girl to the swings. But I had heard enough. I had once again been reminded, by an innocent little girl, all that there is to be thankful for.

I found myself thinking of my friend Miriam. Miriam was always telling me how her grandmother in Israel was almost an invalid. She had trouble with her hip and could barely get off her bed. Her daughter Geneshe, Miriam's aunt, suffered from mild retardation and never married. When Geneshe was born, her mother viewed it as a curse from Heaven. She was heartbroken and could not see any reason for this "curse." Geneshe never attended school and was kept mostly in the house. Still, she had a wonderful disposition and was sweet and friendly with anyone who just took a minute to look at her.

When Miriam's mother married into the family, she observed how her sister-in-law was being ignored and treated like an unwanted piece of furniture. She took immediate action. She did some research and discovered a school for the mentally disabled that would teach her disadvantaged sister-in-law some skills to enable her to join the work force. Not long after, Geneshe landed a job as a teacher's aide in a pre-school, where she was very successful. She continues to hold the job to this day.

As Geneshe's mother became old and ill (she was already in her forties when she gave birth to her youngest daughter), she found her Geneshe was turning into a blessing rather than a curse. Geneshe proved to be indispensable. She was always home to help her mother dress in the morning, take her mother to the doctor or a *simchah*, and hundreds of other little tasks that her elderly mother could no longer do on her own.

If you were to meet Miriam's grandmother and ask her all about her family, she would praise her children and grandchildren as any mother and grandmother would do. But then a small smile would appear on her wrinkled face. "They're all nice and very fine, but Geneshe—she is a blessing from Heaven."

Further away, over at the table near the large tree stump sits Mrs. Schreiber with her daughter, Mashy.

Mrs. Schreiber is also here at Camp HASC to spend the day with her daughter. Mashy, too, has Down's Syndrome, but she got the worse end of the deal. Her IQ is pretty low, and she is very thin and frail looking. Her sister from Lakewood, as well as her other two siblings, one from Monsey and one from Boro Park, have come with their little children to visit her. Mashy is happy to see them all and gives them all a big smile. Now that she no longer lives at home, she still recognizes the various family members but does not call them by their names.

It is late afternoon. The siblings have left, they have a long ride ahead of them, and mother and daughter are alone. I glance in her direction and I smile. Mrs. Schreiber smiles back. "Hi, how do you do?" I was always aware of the wide gaps that exist even among the so-called "mentally retarded." I assume that Mrs. Schreiber knows this and realizes that her daughter is on the bottom of the scale. "No wonder she looks gloomy," I think to myself sympathetically.

The others have gone off in different directions, and I found myself sitting alone. I decided to walk over to this Mrs. Schreiber and make some friendly conversation. Perhaps it would help her pass the time.

"Hi," I said. "In case you don't know, I am Leibish's sister."

"Oh, I keep hearing of Leibish. He is a big shot around here!"

"I guess after coming here for so many years, he feels himself important with his seniority," I reply.

I feel uncomfortable. I have not come over to emphasize Leibish's superiority over Mashy, so I try to downplay it. "Mrs. Schreiber, I hope you don't mind my asking, but is Mashy your daughter or granddaughter?"

"Oh no, she is mine," Mrs. Schreiber answers. She puts her arm around Mashy and holds her close. "If Hashem chose to place Mashy into my family, I thank Him that He has chosen me and not any of my children!"

I nod gently. But Mrs. Schreiber has more to say.

"Don't get me wrong, I love her and never once do I complain, 'Why me?' By looking at Mashy you might get the wrong impression. She is not in the best of health, and you might get a very gloomy picture. I don't want you to get the wrong impression. You have a few minutes?"

"Sure. I am always glad to hear how other families cope with such a child."

Her story did much to change my initial impressions.

For the past few years, Mashy's parents were forced to place her into a home for health reasons. Her heart murmur, with which she was born, has been aggravated by a slow thyroid, a common problem associated with Down's Syndrome. After several emergencies, when Mashy had to be rushed to the hospital, unable to breathe on her own, Mr. and Mrs. Schreiber realized it was in Mashy's best interest to be placed in a home where she could be given special care in controlling her heart and various other ailments she was suffering from.

Still, every *Shabbos* and *Yom Tov* sees Mashy back with her family, happy and content in her own environment. When her van turns the corner of her house, she lets out a "Whoops!" She recognizes that this is her block and soon she will meet her beloved parents.

Mashy must be kept on a very strict diet to control her weight. Even the slightest weight gain could prove hazardous to her health. Starches and fats are a no-no. Mashy loves her mother's home-made *challos* but has learned that it is "bad for her, it could make her very sick." Nevertheless, Mashy sneaks her mother's piece of *challah* while her mother turns her back. All it takes is a few seconds, and when Mrs. Schreiber turns back her *challah* is gone. Mashy has swallowed it quickly and pretends to be looking for it, too.

When Mashy was barely a year old, Mrs. Schreiber, who had just put her to bed for her nap, heard a loud thump coming from the baby's room. She ran in and couldn't believe her eyes. Mashy was sprawled on the floor. There was no one else in the house and she was truly dumfounded. Perhaps she did not put her to bed after all! "I bet I had put her down on the floor to get something from the drawer, and she was so quiet that I left the room thinking she was in bed."

She picked up Mashy, who was still whimpering softly to

herself, and placed her gently into the crib. For some reason, she decided to stay in the room. She did not trust herself. Sure enough, Mashy started to hoist herself up on the railing, and before her astounded mother could think what to do, she had rolled herself over the top and, were it not for Mrs. Schreiber's instinctive reaction, would have fallen to the floor. So her mind wasn't playing tricks, after all. Mrs. Schreiber was delighted with her baby's feat. Maybe she will be an exception? Maybe she will grow up and make history!

As Mashy grew up, she disappointed her parents. She wasn't going to be an exception after all. Although she had an extraordinary ability for climbing all over the house, even climbing up the stairs long before she was able to walk, in most areas her progress was below average. She started to walk some time before her fifth birthday, and her speech was slow to develop. In fact, it is still very limited even to this day, as she approaches her nineteenth birthday.

The Schreibers were never ashamed with their daughter. She was heaped with love and attention from her parents and family. Mrs. Schreiber still recalls how she once went visiting with her family to her brother. Six-year-old Mashy found some blocks, and she started stacking one on top of the other. She clapped her little hands in delight as the blocks climbed higher and higher.

"Shmuli, look," a young voice rang out. "Mashy can play!"

One of her nieces had been watching Mashy and was amazed to see that this "creature," of whom everyone spoke only in whispers, could actually play. Living in Far Rockaway, they had never seen Mashy before and imagined her to be little more than a vegetable.

Mashy was no vegetable, and no one knew this better than

her mother. When Mashy was already three years old, it became increasingly difficult to go for a walk with her. She did not walk, but did not like the carriage, either. If her mother wanted to go right, she "said" left. She had learned to place her feet on the ground, and they acted as very efficient brakes. Mrs. Schreiber could push all she wanted but could not fight those "brakes." She had to relent, and only when she turned in the direction Mashy pulled could she proceed.

When Mrs. Schreiber found herself in the fruit store instead of the grocery and in the hardware store rather than the trimming store, she knew that she had to do something about this. All the fruits and vegetables in the world would not help her when she needed a box of cereal (in those days, fruit stores sold produce and grocery stores sold groceries). The hardware store salesman said sorry, they did not carry three-quarter inch gold buttons.

Mrs. Schreiber decided to enroll Mashy in HASC. While Mashy was away, she could find some time when she could attend to her miscellaneous errands. She still made sure to take her daughter out for walks, but not when she needed anything in particular. Mashy might not have been able to advance academically, but she was a genius in getting her own way.

Despite her low IQ and various ailments, Mashy is a delightful child. She spends the day in a special classroom where she is taught various lessons in self-care and learns to assemble puzzles and to differentiate among colors and shapes. Her mother visits her often, sometimes even twice a day. Her love for her daughter is unimaginable. Whenever she meets a couple with a child who has Down's Syndrome, she eagerly encourages them and reassures them.

"You will see," she tells them warmly. "You will have so much joy from this child. I can tell you from experience!"

Time and time again, I am convinced that Hashem knows to whom to give these exclusive gifts. They are very special to Him, and he must choose their accommodations carefully. They must be valued and treasured.

Right now, as we sit there, the sun slowly following the downward slope of the horizon, Mashy is in another world. She has a small transistor pressed to her ear, and she listens intently to some music. She is adept at finding her favorite stations. She has learned which position on the dial yields the music of her choice.

Even after the others have left, her mother sits with her throughout the afternoon and into the evening, faithfully spending the allotted time with her. Enjoying it.

Presently, I spot Mr. Kahn, and I dash over to him. It is no small feat to catch him with a free moment. Mr. Kahn puts the president of the United States to shame. He is a man who puts in a twenty-five hour day. How? He gets up an hour early.

"Mr. Kahn, you know I'm a 'Curious George,'" I say. "How is Leibish these days?"

I ask it light-heartedly. I've asked these questions before, and I was always gratified. This time is no exception.

"Oh, Mrs. Perkovsky, you should have been here on *Shabbos*. No, not this *Shabbos*, every *Shabbos*."

"How is that?" I ask.

"He steals the show every time. You know we have a little *farbrengen* after the *seudah*. Well, Leibish gets up on the stage, and the kids laugh even before he does or says anything. He has that twinkle in his eyes, as if to say, 'Wait and you'll see what the one and only Leibish has in store for you.'

"First come the *grammen*. Yes, you heard right. He prepares *grammen* before *Shabbos*, HASC style, and reads it off the paper in his hand. You might not believe this, but the *grammen* actually rhyme." (Of course, I do. His sense of humor is so much like my father's, that it makes sense that his *grammen* are also. My father can make up *grammen* faster that you can count 1,2,3—but don't rush.)

"When he has the whole *oilem* in stitches, he becomes serious, takes on a solemn tone and begins his *Dvar Torah*. He has the kids around his thumb. First, they are laughing and giggling with his 'comic strip,' but as he begins the *Dvar Torah*, they become very quiet and listen.

"They can relate to his form and speech, and many can actually understand what he says. It is a revelation to them that 'one of them' can speak about a subject which is usually referred to in such complex terms that they feel shut out. Here they are not only involved but the direct audience. It gives both the performer and the spectators a very positive feeling. Even when one of the staff helps Leibish with the *Dvar Torah*, he insists on wording it his own way. From experience, we find it is in the best interest of everyone concerned to let him have it his way."

Mr. Kahn looked at his watch and exclaimed, "I don't believe this. There is a family waiting for me at my office, and I am a full ten minutes late. Mrs. Perkovsky, you have a special talent. You know how to get me. You know that Leibish is my weak point. How can I be asked about 'the star of the show' and just shrug my shoulder with, 'Oh, Mrs. Perkovsky, meet me at the office and we'll talk?'"

My heart almost bursts. It is a special feeling—not even when my childrens' teachers compliment me about my own children do I feel it. It is unique, a singular sensation one can only appreciate with a unique human being such as my brother.

The children are back from the playgrounds, and the adults

begin to yawn and decide to call it a day. We wave to Leibish, who at this point is as tired as the rest of us. I detect no sadness in him. He was happy to have us come, but he is ready for the farewells. He is an adult who is eager to get back to routine, as we all are.

What is most gratifying is that Leibish enjoys life, particularly when he sees that his whole family comes and when he feels how they all love and care for him. To me, this show of togetherness and the close family ties between us and Leibish is not a tragedy. It is a day of thanksgiving for the good in life, the good in us all.

The Sky is the Limit

▼

Something happened last week, a small incident, but which proves something that people with Down's Syndrome do not level off, that there is no limit to their learning. It is time we realized that no child can be labelled as never going beyond the mental age of seven or ten or twelve. With the proper setting and constant motivation, they can go far beyond anyone's expectations.

Etty, always into the latest inventions, bought a personal computer. Understandably, it has almost taken over the household. There is always someone at it, either typing on the word processor or playing games. If one of my kids is missing, I just have to pick up the phone and dial Etty's number, and *voila*! I have guessed right. Everyone wants to try his hand at the mechanical brain.

Leibish, who is as welcome there as anyone, could also be found in front of the computer, playing along with his nieces and nephews. But there is one program he has never used—the word processor. Whenever he comes, Etty programs the computer to one of his favorite games and the other programs he enjoys. If she is in middle of typing, which she does from time to time for her husband, he looks on, observing her swift fingers moving over the keyboard or, more often, joins the kids in the next room.

This past *Erev Pesach*, she carelessly left her computer on. I say carelessly, because with seven little children around, they could introduce more viruses than any anti-virus can combat. Etty was in the kitchen all morning, cooking, baking and most of all, going crazy. The kids, who had been off from school for most of that week were getting bored. It was raining (why not?), and she was almost at the end of her wits.

She had completely forgotten that Leibish was in the house. Not a hard thing to do. She wished he would give her kids some lessons in behavior. Suddenly, she remembered that she left the computer on and dashed into the room to shut it off.

There, completely engrossed in his work, sat Leibish. He did not even notice her presence. She watched him in wonder as he typed at a pretty good speed many words. "Shop-baby-house-book-enjoy. My name is Leibish. I live at . . ."

There were no spelling mistakes, not one word was repeated, and there were even spaces between each word. After every few words, he would press the return button to start a new line.

She was truly amazed. No one had ever taught him about the space bar nor the return button. He had never typed before, and here he was typing as well as any of her children who have had access to the word processor on a regular basis.

She ran to the phone and dialed my parents' number excitedly. She had to tell them how smart their son was. Of course, my father was not at all surprised. He never is. At least, he never lets on if he is. She felt a little silly. "I should learn to control myself. So what if he types and knows his way around in the computer?" she thought. "If he can deliver all over Boro Park for my brother, if he can work in the warehouse of a supermarket (he has just gotten a part-time job in Pathmark), why shouldn't he know how to press a few buttons on a computer and form words and short sentences?"

Reluctantly, she went back into the kitchen, finished with the *Pesach* preparations and got everyone dressed for the wonderful *Yom Tov* of *Pesach*.

Later that night, as they sat around the *Seder* table waiting for the kids to bring the *afikomen* out of hiding, there was a knock on the door.

Was it Eliyahu Hanavi? Since when does he need to knock? Sruly, the "brave" one, went down to open the door, and lo and behold, it was my parents and Leibish coming to join them for the last part of the *Seder*. What a wonderful surprise! My father, with his lovely voice, and the eager grandchildren, who were very much awake, all joined together to sing those *Pesach* melodies.

Everyone *bentched* and settled back for *Hallel*. My mother signaled to my father that she was tired. They had already finished the *Seder* at home, and so my father got up to go. But Leibish had other ideas. He was not going till we sang *Chad Gadya*. My father has a very amusing version of it, with Yiddish verses mingling with *Lashon Kodesh*, and it is especially enjoyable when it is sung in a crowd.

Well, if Leibish wants something, it is not taken lightly. He makes all kinds of motions and urges his father to, "Please, take it easy. Why are you in a hurry? Sit down and enjoy yourself."

How can one ignore such pleas?

So they stayed on, and Etty claims she has yet to remember such a great time at the *Seder*. Everyone sang, and the atmosphere was truly *derhoiben*. When the *Seder* was over, Leibish was still adamant about staying.

"Tatty, come on, we did not say *Shir Hashirim* yet!" he insisted.

Enough was enough. It was time to put his foot down. "Leibish, remember the *afikomen* you asked for," my father began.

All the kids were curious. They wanted to know what the *afikomen* was going to be. It must be something special if it could persuade Leibish to go home despite the fact that he had not said *Shir Hashirim*.

Sruly guessed it was a watch.

Hilly guessed it was a tape recorder.

Little Fradele guessed it was a pack of gum.

No one guessed that it was a computer.

Yes, Leibish is getting a computer. He is really going places! Etty is proud to have brought this about, and she has already resolved to make a special effort to help him get started. She shall come to the rescue when the keyboard jams, or when a message comes on the screen advising, "Press any key to continue," but the only button that works is the "off" and you continue your knitting instead. She will be glad to obtain some new games and educational programs for him.

But most of all, she will be there, along with the rest of the family, for him. To give him, as he gives us so abundantly, all the love he deserves and to help him reach new and higher goals.

Because with Leibish, the sky is the limit.

Time Out

▼

When parents leave on a vacation, their children see this as an opportunity to visit with friends and spend an extended "pajama party" at their house. The parents enjoy their time away from home, when they can put their concerns on hold and spend a couple of weeks in total enjoyment and relaxation. They can then come back to happy, well-adjusted children who are glad to have had this freedom and yet happy to have their loving parents back.

When the child has Down's Syndrome, the picture takes on a new dimension. The parents, even when they can tear themselves away for a while, find the experience so complex and worrisome that it ends up being anything but a vacation. To begin with, it is hard to find someone to care for this child. And even when someone is willing to babysit, the parents worry constantly. Perhaps it is too hard on them, or perhaps the child will feel homesick and will not be understood when in distress.

For my parents, as long as we were still home, they felt relaxed about going away occasionally for a couple of weeks to Israel or Florida. We knew Leibish well, and he hardly felt their absence. Once we were married, it became increasingly difficult to leave. Where will he stay when they are away? This has become the big question. Raizy? Her girls are bigger now, and things can get complicated. There could be the question of *yichud* if Raizy and her husband have an evening out and leave their girls alone with their uncle. Etty and I have small apartments, and Leibish needs a room to himself where he can feel free to do his own thing. Chavy is presently the best candidate, and she welcomes him gladly.

Her children are very sensitive to Leibish's feelings, especially when they see their parents as well as their aunts and uncles show so much kindness towards him. There is no lesson that will teach a child better than example. "Practice what you preach" is our motto, and Chavy is the first on the bandwagon. My parents appreciate this immensely, and I suspect this contributes greatly to their affection for their daughter-in-law. Chavy sets aside the guest room where Leibish can have all the privacy he wants. His tape recorder and tapes are given a special corner. Last time my parents left to Israel, Leibish stayed with Lezer and Chavy, and he had a great time.

Along with his suitcase came specific instructions: Leibish must be woken up at six-thirty a.m. He must make the *minyan* at Shaar Hatorah, a *shul* that has a hard time with their weekday morning *minyanim*. Many a morning, the members must stand at the corner and almost beg for a "tenth man" for *Shacharis*. Leibish feels very important knowing that he is so indispensable. My father seems more concerned for Leibish to have a good time than for himself. Chavy smiles and assures my parents that they need not worry. Leibish is a big man and will manage just fine. Leibish settles himself in and feels at home immediately.

The first morning, Lezer wakes Leibish up at six-thirty on the dot. It has been many years since the days Lezer shared a room with Leibish, and he had almost forgotten what a job it was to get him to wake up. (Leibish is a very deep sleeper.) Mommy claims that if it was up to him he would have chosen a different time to get up—much later, to be sure. I would not be surprised if sleep is his next favorite pastime after music. Lezer is amazed how machine-like Leibish goes about his morning ritual. It gives him a sense of how many tasks and lessons Leibish must have mastered in his lifetime by the process of habituation. He washes up and gets dressed in precisely fifteen minutes. Every morning he puts on certain articles of clothing first, some last, never varying the pattern. Another five minutes are taken up for a glass of milk. (Don't tell anyone, especially not diet-conscious-Mommy, but Chavy gives him chocolate milk—not that she has a choice. He sits there like a king on his throne and commands sternly, "Nu, Chavy, a glass of chocolate milk!" As if he gets it at home all the time.) He goes about all this in the same unhurried manner. He will not be rushed. Nothing will make him alter his routine.

Before he leaves, he asks for his "breakfast sandwich." Lunch is served at the HASC workshop, so he gets a sandwich to eat for breakfast when he arrives at work directly from *shul*. Knowing the fussy eater he is, Tatty brought home exactly ten rolls (two weeks less two *Shabbasim*). Mommy filled each with a slice of American cheese and wrapped each one carefully in aluminum foil. The sandwiches were then placed in Chavy's freezer. It chokes me up to think how devoted my parents are.

Instead of concentrating on their own packing and travel arrangements, they had Leibish's sandwiches in mind, that, *chas veshalom*, he should not have to eat something he doesn't like.

When the sandwich is safely in his pocket, he asks politely, "My two quarters, please." Leibish gets a special fare discount, and by presenting his bus pass, he pays only fifty cents.

On the third morning, Lezer decided to see what would happen if he gave him five dimes instead.

"Hey, hey, this is not good," Leibish complained. "I need two quarters!"

Here, too, Leibish balks at change (pun unintended). If two quarters is what he always gets, he will not settle for any other form of money.

The final ten minutes of this crucial first half-hour are for travelling. The *shul* is just three blocks away, but Leibish won't walk if he can travel. Anything on wheels, if you please. Some time back, when he first mastered the bus routes in Boro Park, he learned that with the same fifty cents, if he asked for a bus pass, he could take the Forty-ninth Street bus down to Thirteenth Avenue and there change to the Thirteenth Avenue bus down to HASC. Leibish lives closer to the Sixteenth Avenue bus and could reach the school just with one bus. But why take one when you can take two? Sounds complicated? Well, not to Leibish. To him the rules are simple, "Never travel less when you can travel more."

Coming home, Leibish must first unwind. One of the critical roles in Leibish's upbringing was allowing him to unwind in the privacy of his home, while teaching him remarkable control in public. Needless to say, that doesn't mean that at home he can act uncontrolled. Leibish sits at the dinner table with manners fit for a king's banquet. He uses his fork and knife, tucks his napkin into his collar, nobleman fashion. When guests are present, he sits quietly and joins in occasionally in a reserved gentlemanly way.

Yes, I have one word for him, and I am one hundred percent certain that if you were to ask anyone to give you one word that describes him best, the word that would immediately come to mind would be none other than gentleman.

This "anyone" might be his next door neighbor Mr. Berg, a lonely frail man, whom he unfailingly greets every morning with a hearty "Good morning, Mr. Berg."

Or perhaps it might be the woman who just married his second cousin's uncle, who just came to a *simchah* and looks around for anyone whom she might recognize amongst these *tzugekimene* third cousins twice removed. Just when she has given up, and thinks to herself miserably, "No one even knows me here. I should learn not to come if I am not certain there will be any close acquaintances," along comes Leibish with a big smile. "Hi, Mrs. Friedman, how are you?" he says.

Sure enough, some other guests turn around to see who this Mrs. Friedman might be whom Leibish is so happy to meet. They look and see no one they know.

Leibish is not finished. He turns to his sister Raizy. "Hey, Raizy, don't you know who she is?"

Raizy hopes she doesn't blush, but Leibish continues enthusiastically without waiting for an answer. "She just got married to Yitzchak's uncle Mr. Meir Friedman. He had his *sheva berachos* in our *shul.*"

"Oh!" Raizy exclaims with a look of recognition spreading over her face. "Aren't you a Porges girl?"

Mrs. Friedman-nee-Porges and Raizy become engrossed in conversation, a life-long friendship blooming thereof.

Talk about an asset to society!

Once Leibish sees a face, he makes all the connections, will tell you the person's whole family tree and will forever greet them as best friends. He has added much sunshine to people's dreary, cloudy days. In his unassuming manner, he detects an unhappy countenance faster than the best psychologists and will rush to bring cheer and good humor.

Being human and having his special needs, Leibish must have time for himself, where he is not supervised constantly and where he can enjoy himself in his own particular manner. Whereas your every day executive will throw his shoes off when entering his mansion, sit back on his couch, put his feet up on the living room table (for that they need genuine brass?) and turn on the television, Leibish enters his room and turns on the music. He closes the door, as if to keep it all to himself, not to let even one beloved note escape. The side effect being some peace and quiet for everyone else. "How weird," he must think. "They would rather have quiet than this music?"

The quality of the music turns out to be debatable. With two tape recorders and a stereo record player, each playing a different song, one needs courage to call it music. But ask Leibish. He hears each song distinctly and follows them verbatim. He adds another touch to this entertainment. Waving "Buster", his favorite pet (a cuddly little puppet Raizy bought him many years ago) in one hand, while holding his microphone in the other, he sings along joyously, at times dancing until the whole house vibrates.

How lucky he is to have this hobby. This has been going on for most of his life, and it is the best thing that could have happened to him. My parents, in their infinite wisdom, do not restrain him. On the contrary, they approve and encourage it, so long as he doesn't overdo his limits and does not cause any damage. Realizing this, Chavy, too, allows this very necessary "unwinding period."

Supper must be simple. Leibish is a real meat and potatoes man. His opinion about vegetables, "This green stuff is not for me. It looks like grass." What about health? "It's okay. You can have it." A most generous soul. To him, a hearty goulash accompanied by plenty of soda (preferably sweetened) and with his nieces and nephews on either side, is the closest thing to *Gan Eden.*

Coming back from *Minchah-Maariv* finds Leibish a tired man. He has put in his day's work at the workshop, after which he helped out at Shloimy's pharmacy for a couple of hours. For a man with modest ambitions and limited stamina, it has been a long day. His eyes are tired, his movements sluggish.

At ten o'clock, Leibish is ready for bed. The same twenty minutes it takes him to get ready in the morning are now spent getting ready for bed. He prepares himself once again in a steady, unhurried manner and bids everyone good night, a little smile spreading across his gentle face.

"It has been a wonderful day," it seems to say.

A Phenomenal Memory

▼

Wednesday, December 14, 1988

Whenever my family leaves on a *Chol Hamoed* trip, Leibish
is already in the car fifteen minutes before everyone else. He has
a great liking of cars that is surpassed only by music. He
wouldn't mind if we took him around all day by car without even
going anywhere. On the way, he notices every vehicle and could
tell you each name and model, and which person has which car.

When it comes to things that grab his attention, Leibish has
a computer memory. Being a social bug, he takes great interest
in everyone's relations, and when someone is, *chas veshalom,*
ill in somebody's family, he will always remember to ask how
the person feels. We try to reassure him that the person is much
better, even if that is not the case. We just can't stand the look
on his face when he hears bad news. He feels for that person as
if he was his own relative.

Chavy's mother has been very ill lately, and when he
overheard my mother talking with Chavy all about her mother's

201

illness and expressing her regrets that her mother was still not better, Leibish became visibly agitated. It was no use to cover up; he had already heard, and it had upset him deeply. Whenever he meets Chavy's mother on the street, he greets her in such a warm, friendly manner that he has won a special place in her heart. Later, Leibish came over to my mother and said, "What can I do for Chavy's mother that she should feel better?" Like everyone, Leibish needed to know that there was something to be done about a terrible situation, otherwise the helplessness could be overwhelming.

"Well, you can say some *Tehillim* for her," my mother replied. "I'm sure that would help."

Leibish spent the rest of that afternoon saying *Tehillim*, his forehead creased as if he was trying to concentrate as much as possible so that it would be more effective. After that, whenever he saw Chavy he asked her, "How is your mother?"

Chavy knew she must have a positive answer. "She is, *baruch Hashem*, much better."

Relief was spelled all over his face, as if a big burden was lifted off him.

When I think of Leibish's ability to remember and recognize people he has not seen for a long time, there is one incident that immediately comes to my mind.

When Leibish was nine, my parents spent the summer in New Hampshire. We were all married, and Lezer was learning in Eretz Yisrael, so they decided to forego their usual bungalow and spend a summer in New Hampshire. They took two rooms in a boarding house where there was plenty of company for Mommy, and the *shul* was close by for Tatty.

Mommy befriended a woman by the name of Mrs.

Morgenthal. Mrs. Morgenthal was from Washington Heights and was about the same age as my parents. She and her husband were a happy and loving couple, but they had one big void in their lives. They had no children. As the weeks passed, Mrs. Morgenthal fell in love with Leibish. Every morning, he would run over to her and give her a big hug, followed by, "Good Mornig, Mizez Mogento!" The days were long, and Leibish had plenty of time to just sit around with the ladies. They all had a nice word for him and would offer him chocolate and candy. Leibish spent the mornings *davening*, closely supervised by Mommy, and after that he went along with the ladies for the daily half-mile walk. Mommy felt this was a good form of exercise for him.

There are very few activities that Leibish has ever been interested in. Swimming was out of the question; he had terrible aquaphobia (fear of water) and refused to even dip his feet into the shallowest part. The social worker at school felt it was not in his best interest to force him. The fear might be too much of a shock to his heart, and it would end up being more harmful than beneficial. He had no skills at playing the usual games children played, like baseball and basketball. The other children on the block would not play with him. He was far too clumsy, and he had no interest in playing with the younger children who would have agreed to play with him. Somehow, he felt they were not his age and that he would feel out of place with them. In this way, Leibish spent a good part of the day in the ladies' company. He seemed to be content, his need for excitement and stimulation being far less than that of another child of his age.

On a beautiful afternoon, towards the end of August (and the end of the summer), Mommy found herself sitting in the company of Mrs. Morgenthal. They were sitting out on the patio, trying to absorb as much of what remained of the summer's sunshine. Mommy noticed that Mrs. Morgenthal was hemming and hawing until Mommy asked, "Mrs. Morgenthal, you seem to have something up your sleeve. Let's hear what you have to say."

"Well, it's like this." She shifted in her chair uncomfortably and hesitated.

"Don't worry, I will keep it confidential," Mommy said. "Obviously, you want to get something off your chest."

"You are right, Mrs. Weinfeld. I do have something I want to discuss with you. You must have realized that I love your little Leibishl. He is so loving and responsive, he warms my heart. You know that we are childless and have long ago given up having children of our own. We discussed this, and we both agreed that, with your permission, we would adopt Leibish. You already have five healthy children, and I am sure that without Leibish on your hands, you will have more time for yourself. You expressed your desire to take up swimming and some other hobbies you have found difficult to partake in because of your preoccupation with Leibish's many needs. You have already done more than your share with him, and now I feel that perhaps I can take over. I am always running to hospitals and nursing homes, trying to make my stay in this world as fruitful as possible. I always have this guilty conscience that being child-less I have not done my share of good deeds. By adopting Leibish, I will no longer worry that my stay in this world has been in vain."

Mrs. Morgenthal looked at Mommy expectantly, apparently convinced that Mommy would jump at this offer. Here was her chance to give up Leibish to a loving Jewish couple, where he would receive much love and attention. She would not have to fret about having dumped him somewhere in a home where there were no parents for him and where he would be just another number. He would eat kosher and observe the *mitzvos* just as before. She was shocked, therefore, when Mommy answered, her voice proud and resolute.

"You are most kind, Mrs. Morgenthal," she said. "I am certain that you meant every word, and I also know that you would make excellent parents for Leibish. But I am selfish. I want him all to myself. I have grown to love him even more than my other children. I find being away from him even for a little while a wrenching experience. Besides, I am lazy. I don't want to run around to nursing homes and hospitals, and by keeping Leibish near me, and doing everything I can to better his lot, I can have these *mitzvos* right in my home."

Mrs. Morgenthal was deeply disappointed. Her hopes of having a child, and having Leibish would have been even more gratifying, were thwarted. But in spite of her sorrow, she could not help but admire Mommy's courage and unwavering determination.

Years passed, and the incident was all but forgotten. Mommy spent the following summers in the Catskills once again and had never seen Mrs. Morgenthal since. One day, as Leibish was playing outside the dress shop, waving to cars and greeting those he knew, he chanced to see a familiar face. A woman was coming towards him, and she almost passed him by when he called out to her, "Mrs. Morgenthal, you are going away without saying hello to my mother?" She took another look at this "stranger," and suddenly it all came back to her. She embraced him and promised she would go into the store to say hello to his mother.

When Mrs. Morgenthal entered the shop, there were several customers already there, and Mommy was busy helping everyone with their choices. When she looked up and saw someone had just come in, she turned and asked politely, "Yes, can I help you, please?" She had absolutely no idea who this new "customer" was. In New Hampshire, the ladies felt it more comfortable to walk around in their *tichels* and hardly anyone bothered wearing a *shaitel*. In addition, the years had taken their toll. Everyone looked a little older, a little more wrinkled.

Mrs. Morgenthal smiled. "Mrs. Weinfeld, I see you don't recognize me. I will try to refresh your memory. Do you remember someone who wanted to take your Leibish home?"

Mommy immediately recalled who this woman was, and she warmly invited her to join her for a cup of coffee. Over the coffee and some fresh *rugelech*, Mrs. Morgenthal complimented Mommy on the change she has seen in Leibish. She could tell he had made great strides since that summer, and that he had grown into a very polite, well-behaved young lad. They both couldn't get over the fact that neither had recognized the other, and what's more, Mrs. Morgenthal had not recognized Leibish either. Leibish, however, did not forget a face. The *tichel* or *shaitel* did not make a difference. The face remained engraved in his mind forever.

Always a Child

▼

I had been procrastinating for years, but finally I decided it was now or never. Our apartment had to be renovated and expanded if we were to go on living here like civilized human beings. Having, *bli ayin hora*, nine children, the apartment which once seemed so oversized was now way too small. We had bought the house together with my husband's sister when my first baby, Yankele, was only a half year old. My sister-in-law had three children at that time, and we thought it fair that she take the upstairs apartment which had an extra room. For us, the downstairs apartment with its six rooms was more than enough. When we first moved in I thought to myself, "How will we ever fill up so many rooms?"

Looking back now, I wonder how we can manage with so few rooms. I guess everything is relative. It reminds me of a famous Jewish comedian who, in one of his many jokes, relates how he discusses with his friend the theory of relativity. With

207

much consideration and meditation, they sit there in the park for hours and try to come up with an example best describing this weighty subject. One of them finally claps his hands together and exclaims with delight, "Ah! I got it. When you find seven strands of hair in your coffee mug one morning, that is an awful lot of hair. But when you find only seven strands on your head, that is woefully little."

Now that I did not end up in an asylum after the renovation experience, I am certain I never will. Along with the benefit of a newly enlarged home, I have profited by learning that my nerves are made of steel, that nothing will fray them. The truth of the matter is, I have no reason to complain about my contractor. He was unbelievably, painstakingly consistent. He kept to his principles and never varied his routine. He *always* came late, he *always* added to his original price, and he *always* had to do everything over.

Somehow, I am very stubborn and slow to learn. Whenever we made up to meet, I never failed to show up at the appointed hour. His constant tardiness grated on my nerves and made me miserable. When he finally appeared, three days later, he greeted me with such a sweet smile, it could have sweetened a whole urn of coffee. When I had scraped together the amount agreed upon, borrowing and scrimping in the process, I was hit by a price that would have bought me a mansion in the most exclusive Manhattan neighborhood. Mr. Contractor promised to be finished by the end of three months, and sure enough, two years later he proudly announced, "You see, just like I promised. It is all ready!"

Friends and family witnessed my face growing thinner, my forehead creased in a perpetual frown. They comforted me, "That's the way *they* are." The way they pronounced *they* was blood-curdling. They might as well have spoken about the devil.

There was one fortunate aspect to all this. My parents' upstairs tenants had moved out, and the apartment was available for us to move in temporarily. Leibish loved having us so close by, and I had a chance to see him and my parents more often. The kids enjoyed having him around, too. Leibish likes to act the big uncle and when he sees one of them climbing into the garden he admonishes them, his voice conveying authority, "Eh, Eh, where do you think you're going?" My older children look at each other knowingly, as if to say, "Okay, let's pretend we are in awe of him, even though we know that in reality we have outgrown him in every way except age."

I appreciate how they give him the feeling that he is their uncle and has the right to scold them when they misbehave. It is not something I taught them; it is in their nature. When they were little, I did not at first tell them directly about Leibish, I figured they would learn in due time. However, if we came across someone with Down's Syndrome, I would point out, "See, doesn't he look a little like Leibish?" Slowly they realized there was something that set him apart, and they learned to be especially sensitive to his feelings. I did hear my nephew once answer him, "Be quiet. You're not our boss." I called him over and made him apologize for being fresh to his uncle who was older than him and deserved his respect.

They are not embarrassed to walk with him on the street. They feel different from us who grew up with him in one house. I guess being a niece or a nephew is easier. They don't identify with him the way we did. To them, he is only an uncle who, as far as they are concerned, was always around, and that's the way he is. On the other hand, to us he was not always there. For part of our lives there was no one in our family who had a mental disability, and suddenly this person, who is very different arrives and is here to stay. Our world turned upside down, and it took a while to set it right again.

One Friday, while bathing the children, I heard screams coming from the side of the house. I became frightened. I had sent my two oldest boys on some errands, and the first thought that came to my mind was, "Have they been attacked, _chas veshalom_?" I grabbed my little ones out of the tub and threw a towel around them. I called for my daughter to watch them and ran downstairs as fast as possible, dripping water all the way. When I was out the door, I did indeed see my boys, but they, _baruch Hashem_, looked unharmed and were staring in wonder in the direction of my parents' side entrance.

I followed their gaze and beheld Leibish standing outside the door, yelling away. I tried to decipher what he was saying but realized it was no use. When he is collected and in good spirits, his speech is pretty clear, but when he is in distress, he becomes very incoherent and speaks in disjointed sentences. I tried to calm him down while my heart was beating wildly. Finally, I figured out that he was saying over and over, "I can't. I don't feel well. I want to go inside the house." I figured he had lost his keys and was locked out. Instinctively, I put my hand to his forehead to see if he had any temperature, but was relieved to find that he had none. (Thinking back, I realize that subconsciously I do still treat him as a child, just like I do to my own children when they claim they don't feel well. Would I ever put my hand to my other brothers' forehead if they complained they felt ill?)

Just then, I glanced into the house (only the glass storm door was closed) and saw to my amazement that my parents were inside. I saw they did not seem at all perturbed. Apparently this was not so unusual, after all. As I took in the scene, I perceived that the floor had just been washed and that Leibish was to have used the back entrance, something we all did, when we still lived in the house. Leibish kept on wailing, "I must come in through this door (the kitchen). I don't feel well." My parents did not give in. They insisted that he either come in through the back or not at all. They have always used this method with him. Leibish must follow the rules and cannot get away with excuses. It is only by staying firm that they accomplished so much with him, and they must not falter.

Over the years, as Leibish grew up and became a young man, I found myself reassured that he was no longer a child. He was a young man who went to work in the morning, brought home a paycheck at the end of the week and went to *shul* three times a day. This little incident proved to me that although Leibish is an adult and behaves grown-up most of the time, in some ways he is still a child and will most likely remain so all his life.

An Accomplished Detective

▼

"I must get Shloimy. I must get Shloimy. She is a liar. She is a thief!"

Yehudis, Etty's daughter, was walking on the avenue, enjoying a day out in the sun. Just as she started to cross the street, she saw her Uncle Leibish walk past her in great agitation and heard him mumbling these mysterious words.

"Leibish, why are you in such a hurry?" she called to him.

To go on with this story, straight out of Sherlock Holmes, I must introduce you to one of my favorite nieces. Ask Rifkele, Malkele, Raizele and the rest of my nieces (all thirty plus, *bli ayin hora*, not to mention my nephews) and each one will tell you that she is my "favorite niece."

Yehudis is a very friendly sort, mature beyond her seventeen years (listen, ye *shadchanim* out there, wherever you are). She always talks about Leibish with the greatest affection and respect. Yes, you got it. Respect! Just ask her about her feelings about Leibish, and she will tell you. But don't say I didn't warn you. It will take some time. Make sure you got some spare time, brother, because she will give you a very long rundown, which will start something like this:

"First, I must tell you about the time when I went shopping with my friends, when along came Leibish with a big 'hello!' for all of us. After introducing my friends to him, one by one, we stopped to talk.

"As we stood there by the corner, discussing my sister's new baby and my brother's upcoming wedding, a boy of about fifteen, a student at HASC, comes over to Leibish and asks him for a quarter. Leibish says, 'Sorry buddy, I don't have a quarter.' Very patiently, but firmly. Apparently he knows this kid and tries to evade his seemingly inane question.

"The kid does not give up. He repeats in the same monotone, 'Can I have a quarter?'

"This time Leibish is not so patient, but still keeps his cool. 'No, sorry, I don't have,' he replies.

"'Can I have a quarter?'

"Leibish, being only human, has had it by now. 'Hey, kid, do you understand English?'

"'Y-yeah . . .'

"'Then get lost!'

"The kid took off at once."

Then she would go on about his impeccable manners, his warmth and affection. On and on, until she would come to this story about Leibish's mumbling to himself that he must get Shloimy and about some liar or thief.

Yehudis did not like the look on her uncle's face. He was usually very easy going and rarely rushed. He preferred the slow lane. Now, however, he was in a hurry, apparently for some important reason, perhaps an emergency! She decided to follow him.

Two blocks later, they were in Shloimy's pharmacy, which was, as usual, packed with people.

"Shloimy, you must come with me now to the bank!" Leibish exclaimed. "She is a liar! She is a thief!"

Shloimy was clearly amused. "Hey, Leibish, calm down. Yehudis is no liar and no thief. She is a very nice girl."

Leibish, in his distress, was unaware of Yehudis, who had come in right behind him. He didn't realize that Shloimy had mistakenly assumed he was talking about Yehudis.

"Oh yes, she took my twenty dollars from me," Leibish continued. "She said it was no good, but I saw her putting it into her pocket. Sh-she t-took out a torn one from under her desk and s-said th-th-that's the one I gave her. Y-you better come and take it back. Th-they d-don't listen to me, but to you they will."

In his agitation, his speech was very slurred, but Shloimy understood every word. And he was no longer laughing. He turned livid, and after giving his workers some quick instructions, he rushed out with Leibish and Yehudis in tow.

Yehudis's curiosity had peaked by now. She felt like she was inside a detective story, only this was real, with a very interesting cast at that.

They entered the bank, this odd threesome, and went directly to the bank manager.

"Mr. Smith, my brother says a teller of yours just ripped him off for twenty dollars. I know him; he's been doing my deposits for years now, and I have never caught him in a lie. Nor has he ever taken any money or lost any, for that matter."

The manager looked very uncomfortable. He looked around

to see if anyone heard. It would sound terrible for someone to hear that there was a teller in his bank who was pilfering money.

"Mr. Weinfeld, I doubt my teller would do such a thing," said the bank manager. "I bet your brother has miscalculated. Did you check the deposit slip?"

"Yes, I did. I had written five hundred dollars and had counted out twenty-five twenty-dollar bills. The teller crossed out the five hundred dollars and wrote four hundred and eighty. See? Here it is."

Shloimy presented the slip for the bank manager to see.

Mr. Smith became intrigued and, at the same time, alarmed. "Let's go over to the teller and have it out with her." He motioned to Leibish. "Do you remember which teller 'helped' you?"

"Sure I do." Leibish was showing remarkable aplomb.

He walked over to "his" teller's booth. When the teller saw him, she became red as a beet, and suddenly, she became very engrossed in something. Her head was bent low, and she seemed startled when the manager exclaimed, "Miss Lane, please come to the back right now!"

She had no choice but to comply.

Yehudis remained outside the back room where the others had gone in to solve the unpleasant "mystery" which was about to reach its climax. She could hear some loud words, and after a few minutes, they came out, Leibish beaming, Shloimy smiling and the teller crying.

As they made their way back to the store, Shloimy told Yehudis what had taken place inside the back room.

"The teller tried to stick to her story about one of my bills being counterfeit. The manager was eager to believe her. It would be most convenient and would save face for everyone concerned, on the bank's side, of course. But Leibish kept on about the teller having taken his money and having pocketed it.

"The manager soon hit on an idea. He walked over to the teller's desk, and as he felt under her desk, he came across a twenty dollar bill pasted to the underside of the drawer. He had seen enough. He apologized to us and assured us he would discipline the teller."

"Well, you know what the end of the story was?" Yehudis finishes with a touch of drama. She does not wait for an answer, "That teller was disciplined right out of her job. Leibish probably saved lots of people lots of money."

Visit at the Workshop

▼

Recently, I got a chance to observe the workshop, and I was very impressed. My parents were returning from a two-week vacation, and I had offered to meet them at the airport. Tatty requested that I take Leibish along as he knows how Leibish loved a ride, particularly when it involved an airport and airplanes. I called the workshop, saying I would be there at three-thirty to pick up Leibish, and that if I was delayed he should not go home as usual by city bus but should wait for me in the lobby. I did not tell Leibish beforehand, since I did not want his excitement to hinder his performance that day. Like everyone else, being excited causes him to get distracted from the job at hand.

I arrived a little early and decided to go up to the workshop and get a first hand glimpse of the place where Leibish spends half his waking hours. As I climbed the steps, a funny feeling crept through me, in spite of myself. I envisioned a group of

217

sullen, bored employees who would rather be elsewhere. I entered a bit apprehensively and tried not to be noticed. I was pleasantly surprised to observe how wrong I had been to be anxious. The room was alive, with a buzz of activity, and everyone seemed to enjoy his work immensely.

As soon as they noticed me, some of them came over and introduced themselves. Their manners could put many "normal" people to shame. They did not stare at me as if I came from Mars, as happens occasionally when I enter a new place where the people do not know me. They made me feel welcome and at home. I, in turn, introduced myself as Mrs. Perkovsky, Leibish's sister. This was very exciting to them. They had known Leibish for many years and were glad to make my acquaintance. I asked them where Leibish's place was, and they pointed to a table towards the back of the room, explaining that at the moment he was *davening Minchah* in the makeshift *shul* downstairs.

One employee by the name of Sylvia, whom I recognized from the *shul* where my sister Raizy *davens*, was especially friendly. She urged me to come over to her place and inspect her work. She had four stacks of bright, neon-colored papers. Her job was to pick one sheet of each color and place the four sheets into a plastic bag. She proudly displayed her "work-card" in which her daily quota was checked off. I could not really decipher the codes, with which Sylvia was apparently familiar, but I did not want to disappoint her, so I complimented her on her achievement. I asked her if she got along with Leibish, and she hesitated. "Well, lately he is much better," she said at last, "but in the beginning when we wanted to take some of his work, he wouldn't let."

I suggested that maybe he felt they were taking away something that was rightfully his. She explained (obviously she was quite high functioning) that it is the accepted thing to do. When someone runs out of things, they can take from their neighbor's pile. I realized that this place had much to teach Leibish in the field of work ethics and getting along with one's peers.

The staff was very accommodating. They even invited me to come, when I have more time, to get a better picture of how the workshop operates. No one gave me the feeling that I was out of place there. The room has approximately eight to ten tables. Linda is the main supervisor and is responsible for the entire workshop. There are three dedicated supervisors who work under her, each in charge of two to four tables, depending on the work level of the workers. I asked Linda how Leibish was doing, and she was very complimentary. She commented on his sociability, and his improvement, especially his maturity.

I wondered aloud if there was any problem upon which Leibish had to improve. She proceeded to tell me that when Leibish first entered the workshop, he displayed signs of immaturity and was not always cooperative. A few times, out of frustration, he had even thrown things. One time, he wanted a piece of bread at lunch time. He began to yell and proceeded to knock over the bench. At one point, it had become necessary for Shmuel Kahn, the director of the HASC, to go so far as to contact my parents. This was a very rare occurrence. First, Leibish was generally well-behaved, and second, Mr. Kahn did not get excited every time Leibish misbehaved. He understands that everyone is entitled to some bad days, when his mood is less than acceptable. Mr. Kahn has a long, deep-seated respect for the Weinfeld family and the way they handled Leibish over the many years Leibish has been attending HASC. This time they felt it necessary to write a letter in which Mr. Kahn stated that

Leibish was behaving very inappropriately in the workshop. Specifically, he was turning off the lights any time he wished, and he deliberately bumped into the other workers. In the letter, he asked my parents to speak to Leibish regarding his behavior. In addition, they were to sign and return the letter the next day to indicate that they had received it. Sure enough, as was characteristic of my father, he returned the letter the next day, signed and with a little note added at the bottom. "Thank you! We hope that he will behave in the future."

Linda smiled. "We knew that the letter would do it. Leibish loves and respects his parents, and one word of rebuke from them was worth more than any punishment they would have administered. His behavior, thereafter, improved dramatically, and his performance has steadily increased."

So much so, that when a couple of months ago a job opportunity came up at a hardware store in Boro Park, which was seeking a reliable young man who was familiar with the neighborhood, Leibish was chosen above all the others. Among the requirements was that he make local deliveries by foot throughout the Boro Park area and go with the driver and make deliveries throughout Brooklyn. When not out on deliveries, he would have to make sure that all the shelves were clean and neat, unpack boxes and stack items on the shelf. Mr. Kahn and Dr. Wakslak, along with the Director of Vocational Services, Mr. Kenneth Yager, met together, and after extensive review, they decided that Leibish Weinfeld would be the client most suitable for the position. There were two reasons for this conclusion. Firstly, Leibish is a long time Boro Park resident and is familiar with the neighborhood, thereby enabling him to make local deliveries. Moreover, working in the capacity of counselor at the HASC Summer Camp, Kenneth had the opportunity to become familiar with Leibish's neatness and organizational skills; these skills are conducive to proper inventory control and general store appearance. As a result, Leibish was to be interviewed and was excited to seek employment in a competitive work setting.

Presently, Leibish came back from *Minchah*, and I watched from the doorway as he made his way down the hallway towards the workshop. He walked with a resolute, confident step, obviously looking forward to resuming work. On the way, he noticed that the pay phone was off the hook, and he seemed disturbed that someone had been forgetful in replacing the receiver. He replaced it and continued on his way.

I stepped back behind the door so that Leibish should not see me. I loved to surprise him and watch how he reacted. Sure enough, when he finally saw me, delight was written all over his face. "Will you look at that?" he announced ceremoniously for all to hear, while waving his hands dramatically from one side to another. What a great actor Hollywood had missed!

The trip was uneventful, with Leibish having the time of his life. To him, this was as exciting as a ten-day cruise on a luxury liner. It took very little to make him happy. Therein lies his charm. My parents' plane arrived as scheduled, and everyone was happy they were back, most of all Mommy herself. "Nothing beats being home," is all she would comment on the trip.

As it turned out, Leibish began work at the hardware store the following week, spending the mornings at the workshop and the afternoons there, just as arranged. Everyone felt that a gradual transition into the common work force was in Leibish's best interest.

Before long, however, my father called Mr. Kahn and requested that Leibish be reinstated full-time, once again, into the workshop. He explained that Leibish was not being given enough work at the hardware store and spent too much time in idleness. Mr. Kahn welcomed Leibish back and reassured my parents that with his abilities he would find other work very soon.

Obviously, there is still much bias against disabled people, and when a business does hire them, they have very little confidence and underemploy them. We can only hope that, just as there has been tremendous strides in recognizing people like Leibish as an integral part of society, there will be an even greater awareness that they can do much more than previously believed. With this greater awareness will come more job opportunities for the mentally disabled. This will not only provide new chances for them, but also hope and promise for their parents.

Chanala: A Child of Today

▼

Sunday, November 25, 1990

It is amazing how one gains certain perspectives when faced with a problem. At times, there are conditions and situations one never heard of, but when suddenly struck with them, Heaven forbid, one is shocked at how many people are in that same predicament. Over the years, many more families started to keep these children home. It was no longer such a rarity. I was both dismayed at the prevalence of this problem, yet gratified when observing how these loving children have finally found a niche in our society.

I discerned that there were reasons for this new acceptance. Times had changed. People were more willing to travel on new roads and take the untrodden paths. "What will other people say?" went out the window, and with it came greater knowledge and less prejudice. They came to learn that Down's Syndrome was not hereditary, had nothing to do with the parents' genes and was not a reflection on the family nor an obstacle to marrying off the other children. Modern teaching methods, used from very early stages, greatly improved these childrens' development, thus making it considerably easier for the parents to raise them. That is not to say that it is at any time easy, rather, that it is easier.

No one can know for certain, but allow me to go so far as to suggest that my parents indirectly caused many families to take that new path and bring home their handicapped children. Many a mother could have thought, when first discovering her baby's infirmity, "Oh, I just saw the Weinfelds coming home from *shul* last *Shabbos* together with their son who has the same condition as my baby. He greeted me so warmly and the parents looked so comfortable and happy walking with him, surely it can't be as bad as all that." Upon which she calls her husband from the hospital bed and says, tearfully, "Shmuli, I decided to take our baby home. If the Weinfelds can do it, so can I!"

My parents set an example. They proved that keeping such a child was nothing to be ashamed of, that it was through no one's fault and surely not the child's fault that it was born this way. There were some very thoughtless people who made it a point to voice their ridiculous opinions to my parents, such as, "You must have done something in the past that caused this freak baby to be born to you." Or "Maybe the child has a *neshamah* that came down to cleanse itself from some terrible evil it performed in a previous *gilgul*." It makes my blood boil when I recall how insensitive they were to my parents. Fortunately, they were a very small minority. Most people were very tactful and supportive.

The other day, I met Tzivia, my old classmate and good friend. As we often liked to do when we had some time and our children's buses were still a long way off (more than a half hour, an eternity), we reminisced about school and reviewed some of our classmates' present family situations.

"You heard, Simi Ziegelheim just had her tenth child," Tzivia said, her voice a mix of admiration and wonder. "Her oldest is not even eleven!"

"I guess it's still better than not having any children at all. Poor Leah Purvac, she had one pregnancy that ended in miscarriage and nothing since." I winced at the thought.

"What about Esther Katz?" Tzivia asked. "She had six children, a handsome husband, and then boom, a slap in the face."

"You mean Esther Charny, the class leader and head of G.O.?" I asked, concerned. "What do you mean by 'a slap in the face'?"

I always liked Esther, and I used to be very close with her. Before we would leave to camp, we used to take the B train together, down to Mays Department Store on Fulton Street, where we outfitted ourselves in outrageously cheap outfits, perfect for camp's activities. After we both married, we each went our different ways. My husband is a real *litvak*, while Esther's husband, Shloime Katz, is a *heise chassid*. Esther had a hard time persuading her husband to visit her friends; it went against his *shitah*. Gradually, we each met different friends and mingled in different circles. We still held a mutual liking for each other and would greet each other warmly when we met occasionally on the street. Admittedly, I did not see Esther the last five years or so, but I was so busy having and raising my kiddies that I scarcely noticed her absence. Half-consciously I sometimes wondered if she had moved out-of-town, but I never got around to asking anyone about it. Now that I heard that something indeed happened to Esther, I was all ears.

"My sister-in-law lives on her block," Tzivia began, "and she fills me in from time to time. The Katz family has a little girl who seems like a normal child. She plays with the other children on the block, keeping up with many of their activities. But if you look closer, however, you can see that her movements are a little heavier and more sluggish, and sometimes, she has trouble keeping up with the games. Her speech is garbled and unintelligible. In the morning, she gets on a school bus, just like other kids, but her destination is quite different.

"This Chanele, who is now five years old has Down's Syndrome and she's been going to HASC since infancy. It's not like twenty-seven years ago when your brother Leibish was born. Now children with Down's Syndrome, and children with many other mental and physical disabilities, go to special programs where they are stimulated with modern, up-to-date techniques from early infancy. It's called an early intervention and it has brought about tremendous progress. Also, today's parents of such children have a great advantage over parents who had a similar problem around thirty years ago. In those early years, there was no early intervention. There was no place where parents could find relief from the daily hardships when raising mentally disabled children. They had to rely on their own intuition on how to best stimulate and speed up their childrens' progress.

"Babysitters, even when the family could afford it, were scarce, because they did not always welcome working in these homes. Playgroups in those days were rare, and the few that were around were not geared to handle these childrens' special needs. So, the brunt of it, fell on the mothers. All this made these families decide to give up Down's Syndrome children to institutions.

"Esther took all these factors into account and decided, soon after her daughter's birth, to take her home and raise her as part of the family. The adjustment was a difficult one, I hear, but I don't really know the details."

The next day, thinking back to what Tzivia told me about my old friend, I decided to call Esther Katz. I did not look forward to it. All these years I hardly call, and all of a sudden, I remember she exists. How do I begin? However, this ambivalence to call only strengthened my resolve. My father always used to tell us, "How do you know if what you are about to do is a good deed? Look inside your hearts and examine your feelings. Do they urge you to go ahead? If so, stop and give it a second thought— your strong desire is indicative of the *yetzer hora* working on you. When your feelings hold you back and your legs feel heavy so that you find you must make an effort to go ahead with that deed, chances are that it is a *mitzvah* you are about to perform, and the *yetzer hora* is keeping you back with all his might. With experience you will find this rule holds true most of the time." I resolved that my reluctance was a perfect indication that calling Esther was something I must do.

Furthermore, being the sister of a Down's Syndrome child gave me special qualifications. I would be more understanding, and Esther would feel comfortable talking to me about a subject most mothers of such children try to avoid with strangers. At least, this was the case with my mother when Leibish was born. My *yetzer hora* was working overtime. "Forget it, she is probably busy and nervous," the little inner voice said. "She might react negatively to your out-of-the-blue call." I had good reason to suspect that Esther would be busy. First, my friend had told me that little Chanele was the seventh child born to the family, and some more children had been added since. Besides, it was Friday, and who isn't busy on a short winter Friday?

I dialed her number nervously. Presently I heard a voice, a voice bringing back sweet memories of long ago and a longing to be young and carefree once again.

"Hi, who is this please?"

"Take a guess. Remember Fulton Street on a hot June day back . . ."

"Oh, I can't believe this. I bet you I'm dreaming. I'm getting carried away by my imagination. Don't tell me it's Rochel Weinfeld!"

"It's not, it's Rochel Perkovsky, your long lost friend," I said, feeling deliciously sentimental.

For a moment, as we went on talking of old times and the fun we had together on our outings, I wanted to believe that there was no more reason to my calling than to share these wonderful memories of our youth. I was beginning to think that I would leave it at that, that I just called on a whim, remembering our friendship and wanting to relive it once again, now that we were not quite so young anymore.

Surprisingly, Esther changed the subject. She asked me how many children I had, and then I, likewise, asked her the same question, out of convention. I mentioned that I had met Tzivia the day before and she had told me about her special daughter. I knew from experience that to avoid the subject was worse than anything; it was the hardest to take. I told her how Tzivia praised her little girl, how she claimed she looked practically like a normal child. I added that I knew it was a bad time, perhaps I would call her after *Shabbos*. She said it was no problem. She would gladly fill me in on anything I wanted to know.

I think I'll interrupt this story for minute to make an

interesting observation about these special mothers. (I call them special because they have a very special responsibility, which puts them in a very noble and special category.) Over the years, I found they were much more willing to talk about their children than the mothers of a generation ago with the same children. They showed a willingness to share their childrens' development and were gratified to unburden themselves.

"I gather you are talking about my Chanele. Well, she is a very cute and active little girl, but I will not go so far as to say she is one hundred percent normal. Her speech is very unclear, and she is way behind in many aspects. She happened to be very high functioning, right from the start, as early as the first few days in the hospital."

"How could you tell she was high functioning?" I asked.

"When still in the hospital, she picked up her head and looked around and generally was pretty alert," Esther answered.

"How did your family react to her?" I always asked this question first. I found this the key to the whole adjustment process. My cousin in Monroe, who three years ago gave birth to a little girl with Down's Syndrome claims she was only able to cope because of the tremendous encouragement from her children. Most notable were her two oldest kids' responses when first told of their new baby sister's condition.

"Hello, Shloimele, how are you?"

"Fine, Mommy, and you? I miss you!" Being away in Canada for months at a stretch is the culprit.

"Eh, Eh, Ehem . . . we have a *mazel tov* in the family. You got a new sister yesterday."

"Oh, Mommy, that's so exciting. *Mazel tov!* It was about time we had another girl. Seven boys to two girls was a little lopsided, even from a boy's point of view—but you sound funny, somehow, not as excited as usual."

"Well, to tell you the truth, things have not been going too well with the baby. The doctors say she has Down's Syndrome. Do you know what that is?"

Pause.

Quickened pulse, gulp-gulp-gulp, skipped heart beat. "Shloimele, are you there?"

"Y-y-yes, Mommy, of course I'm here. You say Down's Syndrome? The family that invites me sometimes for the Friday night *seudah*, the Brauns, have such a child. She is adorable. You can't help loving her. Whenever I enter the house, she runs towards me and puts her little arms around me and shouts gleefully, 'Shoimy, Shoimy!' And Mr. Rosenfeld brings his nine-year-old Down's Syndrome son Duvi to *shul* every *Shabbos*. You should see how well behaved he is. He even *davens* from a *siddur*."

"Shloimy, I know, I know, but don't you realize that you are a *chasan bachur*? You are sixteen years old already. The way boys get married these days, in a couple of years people will start *redding shidduchim* and what will they think when they hear you have such a sister? Even if the *shadchanim* are intelligent enough and understand that it is not hereditary, that with your *maalos* and *yichus* it is just a side issue, what about the girl herself? She may think 'Well, I realize he is a wonderful catch, but I am not ready to become involved with such a sister-in-law. Let me wait for a more 'normal' *shidduch*.'"

"Mommy, one thing I can tell you, and I hope you will listen and agree. Any girl who does not want me because of *my* little sister, whom I already love without even seeing her yet, I wouldn't want anyway."

Friend, do you know what pride is? I'm afraid not, if you did not see my cousin's face that moment.

Next came the call to her second child, her eldest daughter Tzipporah. Earlier that day her husband had called her to camp (it was the middle of July).

"Hello, Tzipporah, this is Tatty. Mommy had a baby, but there is something wrong with her."

"What's the matter, Tatty?" she asked, concerned. She could hear her father crying and she got really frightened. "Please, Tatty tell me quickly what happened!"

"Tzipporah, I can't go on. Wait for Mommy to call you."

My cousin hung up, unable to contend with this whole business of notifying his daughter about something he himself had not come to terms with.

"Tzipporah, this is Mommy speaking. Has Tatty called?"

"Yes, Mommy, he called this afternoon, and I am still all shook up. I'm imagining all kinds of things. It's awful."

"Well, there is no need to imagine, there is plenty going on right here in real life. The baby was born last night, and the doctors say she has Down's Syndrome."

"What's that?"

This was terrible. Down's Syndrome was a new word to this fourteen-year-old girl, whose main language was Yiddish, and who only knew that such children were "funny," or "a little different." Her alarm intensified at hearing this strange term.

"Well, you know the Frieds who live around the corner from us. They have a girl who is . . ."

"You mean Yitty? The one who runs into the other kids with her tricycle and disrupts our board games when I'm over at her house playing with her older sister Shprintzy? She hardly speaks but giggles a lot."

"You got it."

"Oh, Mommy, I'm so relieved, I thought it was much worse."

"How worse?"

"Well, I thought she was missing a hand or a foot."

Talk about relief.

Esther Katz's story was in a way so similar to my cousin's and some other wonderful women I have met, that I saw some patterns emerge.

Often, the husbands had a harder time coping, leaving their wives to contend with a double problem.

The children were all-accepting, a true blessing.

The first few weeks were the hardest.

The immediate reaction was, "Let's give it up."

Foremost on their minds when deciding to keep the child was, "By no means will we let this child adversely affect our other children. We will do anything for this child so long as it does not disrupt our normal routine."

It so happened that within the decade preceding Chanele's birth, the Katz family had lost both sets of parents. There was no parent on either side to turn to for some much needed solace. Mr. Katz went into a deep depression.

"Can you describe his reaction more in detail, please?" I asked cautiously.

"When my husband found out what was wrong with the baby, he refused to look at her, refused to have absolutely anything to do with her. He would hear of nothing less than giving her away permanently. Even when he picked up the baby at the hospital and kissed her, at the nurse's bidding, he went about it in a mechanical way, much as if he would have kissed our two-year-old daughter's doll. On *Erev Shabbos*, when the time came to decide on a name to give at the *Kiddush*, he protested vehemently against using any of our close ancestors' names. His mother had died only the year before, and he had hoped to have a daughter to name after her. No other grand-daughter had been born since. But this was different. He could not have this "less than perfect human being" named after his dear mother. We finally came to a decision. She would be named after my great-great-grandmother Chana.

"I spent the following two weeks in Sea Gate, the convales-cent home for new mothers and their newborn babies. I stayed in my room most of the time. It was a very uncomfortable feeling to sit together with the other mothers, blissfully nursing and caring for their newborns, while my baby was deposited with a *frum* woman named Mrs. Gottesman in Lakewood, New Jersey, who took in such children until permanent homes were found for them.

"I made my intentions clear. I would take my baby home as soon as possible. My husband never came to visit me. We were in total disagreement. My misery was complete. I had no baby and no husband; things were very unfair. Furthermore, I felt extremely guilty giving up my baby. My conscience ate at me so, that I hired a taxi and travelled to a rabbi who lived not too far from the convalescent home.

"I explained the situation to him, that my husband refuses to have our baby in the house. I wept when I described how, for the past weeks, he had been neither a husband nor a father. My girls had complained to me on the phone that he did not even leave the house except to go to *shul* and to work. If there was a phone call for him, he instructed everyone to say he was not available. The rabbi observed that *shalom bayis* came first, and he advised me to give up my baby, at least temporarily."

There was a knock on the door at Esther's house, and she asked if I could hold on. As I waited for her to come back, I was relieved to hear how the rabbi responded. Judging the situation, the rabbi's reaction was a wise one, or at least understandable. I was reminded of a woman in Queens who told me about her visit to a marriage counselor that turned out to be very disappointing. I had called her to say that I was planning to publish some work on Down's Syndrome and would like to know if she could answer some questions for me. Her response was a very positive and gratifying one. She said she appreciated that someone in our community was willing to give some time and effort to bring this issue out into the open for all to see, to bring it out of the closet where it has been for so long.

When I asked her how she got over her depression, she said, "I am still depressed, but I am learning to adjust." She, too, had for her own personal reasons decided to give up her child, and she went to a certain marriage counselor for advice. His answer was so shocking, it enraged her into a determination quite the opposite of his intentions.

I will not elaborate on what he said. It is so unbelievable that people will say just that "it is unbelievable." Maybe. Let us not believe it and so we do not have to deal with the guilt. But I feel it my duty to relate this first-hand report and leave it up to you to make your own judgment. One more point before I continue with this unpleasant account. I promise to follow it by a very positive reaction of a notable man, who, I'm sure, was not alone in his convictions. There were and there are many other Jewish authorities who have shown enormous sensitivity and understanding for these special children.

Here is this marriage counselor's reply verbatim, per Mrs. Queens. "I believe that these children are somewhere between animal and man, that to bring them home would result in lifelong misery (*tzaros*) and that such so-called 'children' do not belong in a normal home."

I had quickly called my mother and told her what I'd just been told, hoping to hear it wasn't true. It couldn't be! Sure enough, my mother disbelieved it one hundred percent. She added reassuringly, "Do you remember the story with the Satmar Rebbe back in Europe?"

Did I remember! It still warms my heart when I am reminded how the noble and honored Satmar Rebbe *zatzal* went against the tide to protect a mongoloid. (How I hate this term! Surely, you have noticed that somewhere along this book I switched from mongoloid to Down's Syndrome as soon as I learned of this more medically correct term. Now there is even a better term, coined by a child affected by this syndrome who has become a nationally celebrated actor. "I don't have Down's Syndrome. I have Up Syndrome!")

A certain Mr. Klein, a very wealthy Jew from Budapest, came to the Satmar Rebbe and stated, "My wife just gave birth to a baby boy, and the doctors diagnosed it as a mongoloid."

The Satmar Rebbe extended his sympathy and started encouraging the man to have *bitachon* that Hashem would see him through this misfortune. As was his custom, he offered whatever help he could give and promised that he would welcome this baby boy as a beloved member of his congregation.

Mr. Klein shook his head. "No, Rebbe, you cannot help me," he said. "I have decided not to take this child home and to place it in a well-established institution where he will get the best treatment available anywhere. I will not spare any expense to insure that he will be well attended to. I have come to you for a *berachah* in implementing my decision."

The Rebbe's face stiffened. Gone was his usual sweet smile. His voice rose as he exclaimed firmly, "No, I will not give you my blessing. The decision is yours. I cannot force you to change your mind. This I will say. This child has been born with a special *mazel*, 'Shomer Pesayim Hashem.' If you go ahead and give up this innocent child, I can guarantee that you will lose all your wealth and you will never enjoy a good day!"

Needless to say, Mr. Klein was full of remorse when he recognized what a terrible step he was about to take. He begged the Rebbe to help him, and he promised he would take the child home and, with the Rebbe's guidance, would raise him in the best manner possible.

My mother also reminded me of a recent *shiur* given by a certain *rav* that we both attended. The *rav* advised the congregants that they must be aware that when a child is placed in a gentile institution when it is possible to raise it at home, albeit with some inconveniences, they must accept the terrible consequences. Every time this child eats *treifos*, every time the child is *mechalel Shabbos*, every time the child eats *chametz* while his family sits around the *Seder* table, the parents are responsible and will be judged as if they themselves transgressed each time.

Needless to say, there are times when a child is born so handicapped, or when the family really cannot handle it, that keeping it would be far more damaging to the family and the child than beneficial. Each case is unique and must be dealt with as such. The *rav* was referring to parents who relinquish custody of these "less than perfect babies" for superficial reasons, such as for saving appearances or when they are not willing to give up their hitherto trouble-free lifestyles.

Presently, Esther Katz came back to the phone and continued her story, unaware of my thoughts. "The rabbi's words gave me the right, so to speak, to give up little Chanele, and I realized there was no other choice. By saving Chanele, I would be disposing of the rest of my family. It did little, however, to relieve my guilt feelings, and I held tenaciously to my hopes that in time my husband would soften up, would come out of his terrible depression and would allow our child, our flesh and blood, to rejoin our family, where she rightfully belonged.

"As *Pesach* came closer, two events took place that finally brought my baby back to me. When Chanele was four weeks old, Mrs. Gottesman called, saying that she had taken the baby to the pediatrician for a routine check-up, and the doctor discovered a heart murmur. This was not very surprising. It is a common disorder associated with Down's Syndrome. The doctor advised that the baby be taken to a heart specialist. Mrs. Gottesman asked that, since she was tied down with the other babies, some her own and two other foster children, perhaps I could take her to the specialist.

"I took Chanele to a doctor in Manhattan. I got to be with her for a full day and got a good look at this baby whom I hardly knew. I had expected the feelings towards her to be all-encompassing. I was very disappointed. There was something lacking. I held her, fed her and took care of her much as I would have done any of my other children, but my heart was numb. I told myself that this was because we were torn apart right from the start and were deprived of that special bonding that takes place the first few weeks of a baby's life. It plays an important role, in those first and crucial weeks of her life, as it links mother and child into an everlasting love no one else can share."

She continued speaking. "The specialist confirmed that it was a heart murmur but asserted that it was 'innocent.' She would outgrow it in time, and no treatment was necessary. 'Take her home and enjoy her, she looks very alert,' he said. His words stabbed at my heart.

"I did not take her home. My husband still held fast to his 'give it up' attitude. Another two weeks passed, and Mrs. Gottesman called again, 'Mrs. Katz, I'm sorry but I cannot manage it any longer,' she said. 'Another child has been brought to me, much more handicapped than Chanele, and with *Pesach* fast approaching, I must ask you to take her home.'

"I saw my husband looking at me intently, thinking I was unaware he was sitting in the next room on the couch. I took a different tactic. 'Please give me a few more days so that I can find her a new home,' I begged Mrs. Gottesman. I wanted to show my husband that I was trying to place her in another home, all the while intending to bring her and keep her in our home forever, lest what remained of my motherly feeling to her would be crushed and frozen forever. Mrs. Gottesman agreed to give me two more weeks. I made a decision. My husband being within earshot, I would pretend to call up many people imploring them to take in this child whose own parents would not. I took out all the phone books, making sure my husband saw and heard everything. I scribbled down countless 'numbers' and dialed and spoke (to no one in particular. Shakespeare's soliloquies could have taken a backseat to my performance) begging, imploring them to, 'Please, take pity. Accept my child into your home.'

"One conversation went like this. 'Excuse me, you say you have seven other children? Oh, but what would another child matter? She is well behaved and sleeps through the night . . . you ask what reason I have to give up this baby? To tell you the truth, I am deeply saddened about this whole thing. I cannot sleep nor eat, and my life has been one big misery ever since my baby was born. My conscience doesn't give me one moment's peace. I cry and cry some more, but my husband is firmly against keeping her. I have six other children to think of, and unfortunately, the baby must be sacrificed.' I wiped away tears. They were not part of my performance; they were real, bitter tears.

"I hung up, drained but optimistic that surely my husband would be moved. I was right. The fact is, my husband is a loving and devoted man. He will do anything for me and the children. I suspect, although he has refused to discuss it, that this whole matter of refusing to accept Chanele had something to do with this fierce commitment to his family. He did not want to hurt his wife and children by having them deal on a daily basis with it. My phony conversations made him realize how misguided he had been, that he was hurting me far more than protecting me. He agreed to take Chanele home, and she has been with us ever since."

I was completely taken in by this new-found friend. What a wonderful, sensitive woman! What courage and perseverance!

I pressed on. "How does your husband feel towards this special daughter?" I was heartened by Esther's straightforward narrative and pushed on, albeit discreetly, so as not to touch on a raw nerve, not a small feat when dealing with a subject as sensitive as this.

"To say he is close to her would be exaggerating," Esther replied. "In the beginning, he practically ignored her. He busied himself with the other children and somehow managed to stay out of her way. As time passed, and my husband came to see how affectionate and loving she was, he gradually came to accept her more and more." She proudly proceeded to tell me some of Chanele's "*chachmos*." These newfound skills and her fun-loving nature (her first abstract words were "This is much fun!") drew her closer to her father in spite of himself.

The first song she learned to sing was "*Vesain Banu*." Her voice would rise to a pitch, and she would pucker up her forehead in great concentration, clapping her pudgy little hands. When her father, who had hitherto refrained from getting too close, witnessed this "miracle"—that this "different" child was not so different after all—he broke out in a wide smile. Though he didn't say anything, he picked little Chanele up and swung her high in the air. The expression on his face said it all, "I am coming to the realization that you are a child like other children. You like to show off and are learning much the same as anyone else, and I love you for it."

That evening, when they were retiring for the night, Mr. Katz turned to his wife. "You know, Esther, Chanele is quite pretty," he said. "Her hair has grown in and with her neat little features she looks quite attractive. I can't believe how she has developed." Esther smiled and nodded her head in approval. She did not dwell on the subject. She felt there was no reason to push it. Her husband was coming around. He was getting attached to his little daughter and she did not want to interfere.

Once, when the dressmaker came to their house, little Chanele and her two older sisters were told to try on the new dresses being sewn for the upcoming wedding of their oldest brother. The older sisters were reluctant. "How many times do we have to try on these dresses?" ten-year-old Devorah complained. Nechama, the eighteen-year-old *kallah moid*, had just come home from work and made it very clear that she was in no mood for yet another fitting. Only Chanele was cooperative. She eagerly got out of her skirt and pullover. She was proud to show off her ability to undress by herself. She was just as eager to put on her new dress. She looked at herself in the mirror and turning to the dressmaker exclaimed happily, "Yipee, I love new dress. Thank you, lady!" Chanele had just found a new friend. The dressmaker picked her up and planted a big kiss on her cheek. She complimented Esther on raising such a well-mannered little girl. (She had no comment for the older ones.)

We were so engrossed in our conversation, that we did not even realize how late it had become. The kids were back from school, and there was still much to do. I thanked Esther for sharing with me so much about her life with Chanele. I had called to offer support and, instead, found her giving me *chizuk*.

The HASC Concert

▼

Sunday, February 10, 1991

"Rochel, how would you like to come along to a concert?" Raizy said to me one fine day while we were speaking on the phone. "Yittel, Devoiry and I have decided to have a swing at it."

"Oh, I'd love to," I enthused. "Where is it? When is it? Who will be performing? And one more little question. How much is it?"

I looked forward to getting a chance to listen to the "music greats" sing and perform live on stage. Record players and tape recorders have done much to bring music into our homes. The newest stereo systems, disks and the many sophisticated instruments have enhanced the sound quality immensely. I can peel potatoes for the *kugel*, iron my husband's shirts and still have music as close as the nearest sound system.

I can close my eyes and, in the confines of my home, pretend I am in front of a magnificent stage with an enormous orchestra conducted by the most famous conductors. Music is as at home in my kitchen as are my pots and pans. The difference is the sound. I guess I am a little weird, but I prefer music to the pots and pans "conducted" by my little Moishy.

With all our technology, nothing beats live music.

Raizy was asking impatiently, and not for the first time, either. "How much is what?"

"The ticket," I replied. "What else?"

"Well, you can pay one thousand dollars and sit up in the balcony along with the other benefactors," she informed me. "You can pay five hundred dollars and sit up front. Or you can pay one hundred dollars and sit towards the back."

"Are you kidding me?" I said. "One hundred dollars to sit in the back? I might as well stay home and listen to the tape. At least at home I can stretch out on my couch."

"Rochel, you're only kidding yourself. You know you never have time to sit on your couch. You only bought it because Sears had a sale. Little did you realize that Sears products are always on sale."

"Are you trying to tell me that I could have gotten it anytime for that price?"

"You know, Rochel, I didn't call to discuss couches and Sears' sales," Raizy continued. "I better tell you about the concert before I forget. The tickets are going like hot cakes, and if I don't go out to buy them by the end of this week, they will have all been sold out."

"Forget it, Raizy. I am not paying one hundred dollars for any concert. No singer will get me to pay this kind of money."

"Hold on, Rochel. What about your other questions? They are waiting patiently in the corner to be answered. I will reward their patience by answering them in the order you asked. Where is it? It's in Avery Fisher Hall. Who is singing? Abe Rotenberg, the D'veykus group, Mordechai Ben David and the London School of Jewish Song."

"Ohhh, why didn't you say so! Raizy, you know how I love to hear these guys. And you know how I love those little British (I rolled my R for special effects) *yingelach*! Of course, I'll go. But . . ."

"Oh, what is it now?" she asked, exasperated.

"I—I hope my guilt feelings of spending so much money for one evening's entertainment don't spoil it for me."

"I have a way of wiping those guilt feelings of yours off the map," she said.

"Try me!" I challenged. Guilt feelings thrive on me like mold on a soggy piece of old bread.

"What if I tell you that all the proceeds of this concert go to the Camp HASC program? What if I tell you that Leibish has been picked to go on stage?"

I didn't need to hear more. I had heard enough. One hundred dollars seemed very little all of a sudden.

"Raizy, run out now and buy those tickets!"

It was imperative that we not miss this great event. All those great performers (Leibish in particular) and for such a cause! I could not think of a better one. Camp HASC encompasses so many causes, it would be unfair to put it all under one heading. It is special education, caring for the sick and the disabled, providing homes for the needy. The list is endless. It is far more than "just another camp." I couldn't wait to go and be part of this special event for the special children of the Jewish people.

We made up to leave at seven o'clock sharp. I couldn't see how I would ever make it out of the house. Suddenly, everyone was thirsty and everyone had something very important to say.

"Mommy, don't forget to turn the tape over to the other side when the first side is finished."

"Mommy, please check the tape recorder batteries from time to time."

"Mommy, please try not to talk while they're singing."

I needed to be fair. I am against broken promises. How could I promise not to talk when I was going to sit next to Chavy? Chavy reminds me of the motorized car my kids got for *Chanukah*. The difference is, I don't think anyone has located the "off" switch. But I don't mind. Knowing her, she will add to the fun.

Leibish adds to the fun, too. For weeks before the concert, every time we met, he would ask, "Nu, Rochel you got the tickets already? You better hurry up, Mordechai Ben David will be there!" His excitement is contagious.

The horn sounded at seven o'clock sharp. I grabbed the tape recorder and was out of the door. I did not risk looking back; I was afraid. The little ones were not at all happy I was leaving. I did not want them to see how very happy I was to be leaving.

Leibish was already sitting in the car when I came down.

"Hello, Rochelle. How are you?" he greeted me.

Leibish was ecstatic. He was in seventh heaven. The big day had finally arrived.

"Fine, Leibish," I returned. "And how are you?"

I always make sure to acknowledge his greetings.

As I took my seat next to Leibish, a scene flashed before my eyes. I tried to wipe it away, as it threatened to wash away my pleasure with this outing. I did not succeed. The scene presented itself in full color.

Mommy loves to go to *shul* on *Shabbos* and *Yom Tov*. Tatty is the *baal tefilah* at *Shachris*, and Mommy will not miss it for anything in the world. I also love hearing my father's *davening*, as does everyone else, especially the ladies. Sometimes on *Yom Tov*, I make it in time to hear my father finishing the loud *Shemoneh Esrei*, and I enjoy every minute of it. He articulates every word and has a delightfully pleasant and clear voice.

Sometimes, at the end of *davening*, Leibish comes up to the ladies' section. There is a special lady whom he comes to salute. The women are busy greeting each other (there is no talking in my parents' *shul* during *davening*—no *chachmos*!) and wishing one another *a Gutten Shabbos*.

This particular *Shabbos* found Leibish directly in front of Mrs. Ingleman. Mrs. Ingleman, in turn, was directly in front of my mother but was unaware that my mother was in back of her. Leibish, who had come up to wish his mother *a Gutten Shabbos*, did not ignore Mrs. Ingleman. He bowed down to her in his best gentlemanly way and said pleasantly, "*Gut Shabbos*, Mrs. Ingleman. How are you?"

"Go away! Go away!" she replied harshly. "Don't bother me!"

"W-why should I go away?" Leibish stammered, shocked at her reaction. "W-what did I do wrong?"

Mommy was beside herself. She was so enraged with this Mrs. Ingleman, she had to physically control herself from pouncing on her. This same person who was so sweet to Leibish in his mother's presence, was showing her true colors. She had been unaware that my mother was in back of her, and therefore allowed herself to be as rude to this "*meshugene*" as she really felt all along, while outwardly putting on a "nice" front.

My mother decided to use a different "weapon."

"*Gut Shabbos*, Leibishl, how are you?" she said. "It is so

nice of you to come and say *Gut Shabbos* to me. Just go ahead and greet the other ladies. Everyone else is nice, you'll see."

My mother was not about to let this insensitive woman hurt her son.

At this point, as they were making their way out of the *shul*, Mommy found herself face to face with Mrs. Ingleman. She stared hard at her, not saying a word. Mrs. Ingleman felt very uncomfortable, and she would have loved to sink deep down somewhere, out of everyone's sight. Many people had witnessed what happened, and they were not about to let her get away with it. They gave her the cold shoulder and kept away from her as from a vampire.

Leibish soon forgot about Mrs. Ingleman. The other ladies all acknowledged his greetings with love and affection. They had seen him grow from an ambivalent little child into a true gentleman, and they were proud of him.

"You're happy to come to the concert?" I asked Leibish.

He had not seen the "scene" in my mind. He was unaware of my morbid thoughts and was in excellent spirits. The concert took up all his thoughts, as they should have mine. I was glad to be rid of my unpleasant memories and once again to concentrate on the event that lay before us.

"Were you ready in time?" I asked. As if I didn't know.

Raizy laughed. "You bet! He's been in the car since six. He feels that if he sits in the car, the concert will start earlier."

We stopped to pick up Yittel and Devoiry. Now we were all in the car. Chavy with her doggy bag (Chavy must have food with her—it is her security blanket), Yittel with her latest, updated binoculars the better to see the "stars" who would otherwise appear from our seats as remote galaxies—tiny specks in the universe, and Devoiry, unburdened by anything more than her dainty little pocket-book.

We all chattered and giggled, paying very little attention to the road. Raizy, who was the driver, did pay some attention. She stopped at the red lights, kept to our lane most of the time and pretty much followed the directions Mordechai had given her. At one point, Raizy warned us not to distract her. Coming out of the Battery Tunnel, she would have to make a right and "follow the traffic." Mordechai had wisely recommended "not to take her eyes off the road, otherwise she would easily wander off the main street into Heaven only knew where."

Raizy did just that. She kept her eyes intently on the road, but her mind was intently on our animated conversation. We were discussing the pros and cons of war in the charged Persian Gulf zone. The discussion got so heated, it felt as if we were in the Saudi desert, sitting across from Saddam Hussein, who was very interested in our views.

"Raizy, you are going the wrong way on a one way street!" Leibish exclaimed. "Raizy, get off the road, you are going the wrong way. Look at that car! It is coming this way."

The car ahead was flashing its headlights in a desperate attempt to warn us of imminent danger. The danger was not lurking behind bushes or around corners. It was right there, out in the open. There was no mistaking it.

Raizy pulled off the road just in time. Leibish had been on the alert, ready to protect the "adults" who were acting more like the children they had left behind. That was the problem. Unconsciously, we rely on Leibish to remind us when we are turning into the wrong street or when we drive above the speed limit. If I added up all the tickets he has saved us over the years, they would amount to a small fortune.

As soon as we were off the road, Raizy asked if we minded if she stopped for a couple of minutes to collect herself. We obliged gladly. We were all shaken and needed a break.

It was hard to imagine that it was actually winter. Although it was January, the heart of the winter season, the weather was unusually mild on that Sunday, the day of the concert. But our spirits were far from mild. We were as excited as a bunch of kids on their first night out. We were away from the little ones, away from the noise, the uproar, the tumult and the chaos.

Not that the streets in Manhattan were quiet. Not by a long shot. As we walked from our car up Fifth Avenue to Avery Fisher Hall there were mobs of people. Everyone was out to have a good time.

We checked our coats and entered the beautiful arena where the concert was going to take place. Leibish, independent as he is, waved good-bye to us and was off to the V.I.P. section.

Raizy had promised Tatty to look after Leibish. My father hasn't changed. He is still as overprotective of Leibish as ever.

"Leibish, you're sure you know where you sit?" she asked.

"Don't worry, Raizy. I know."

"Have fun, Leibish."

"You, too!"

He did not need anyone to usher him to his seat. Somehow, he knew where to go. I did not even ask him, I knew he would get offended.

Mommy knows he doesn't like when she asks about his comings and goings. But he is her *mezinikel,* and so after worrying an entire Sunday afternoon, she would ask, "Where have you been, Leibish? We were looking for you!"

"What do you mean, you were looking for me?" Leibish would respond. "Don't you know I work for Shloimy? Do I ask where Mommy is (we speak to our parents in third person) when she goes shopping? Or where Tatty is when he is at work?"

He is right. He is not a child anymore, and it is time we trusted him and gave him more credit. He has been travelling independently for years, has walked practically every street in Boro Park and some parts of Flatbush, and it's time we learned that he is his own person, living his own life.

We took our seats and sat back, totally relaxed.

"Chavy, when was the last time you had a chance to sit back with absolutely nothing to do?"

Chavy agreed. It was already paying off.

The concert itself was a smashing hit. The performers all outdid themselves and proved once again that there is tremendous talent amongst us *frum* Jews. I must admit I am also to be blamed for stereotyping us *heimishe* as devoid of any substantial talents. True, there are those that are artistically inclined and can sing and play instruments, I reasoned, but true talent, was only amongst the gentiles and the secular Jews. They can learn in the universities and get a chance to attend schools specializing in the myriad forms of the arts, thus getting the opportunity to develop their inborn talents and expand them.

But over the years, as I looked around me and absorbed our culture, and now as I sat there mesmerized by the fine music and the splendid singing, I have realized how wrong I had been. There is as much talent and as many gifted persons amongst us as amongst any other sect. Maybe more. They are not distorted by an obnoxious society. They do not originate from the drug addicts and drunkards. Rather, they spring forth from pure, untainted sources, complemented by Torah and holiness.

Group after group, singer after singer, each filled the hall with lovely notes and poignant song. I had come to enjoy a night out, while supporting Camp HASC at the same time. I was getting more than I had counted on, far more.

Then came the "beginning of the end." The music took on momentum, and everyone waited expectantly for this final scene. Who, of all the renowned celebrities, would be the one to highlight the occasion?

Would it be Mordechai Ben David, who has gained world-wide recognition as one of the greatest singers of modern times?

Would it be the adorable children of the London School of Jewish Song, conducted and orchestrated by one of the nicest guys in show business, Yigal Calek? They surely would be the topping on the cake, the cherry on top (pronounced "tup")!

We waited and sat there, guessing. Yittel claimed it would be Mordechai Ben David. He still got the loudest applause. If I know her with her binoculars, she might have even taken a count at each applause. Devoiry wouldn't comment. Chavy guessed it would be the British bunch. "I have never ever heard such a moving version of *Hamalach Hagoel*." The way Yigal held the smallest of the group (no more than six or seven years old) on his lap and swayed to and fro with his charges while chanting this age-old ballad, stole her heart. I, for one, could not come to a decision and decided I would wait and let myself be surprised. I hoped it would be something that would leave a good taste in my mouth. Something that would have me come back again and again, year after year.

The lights began to blink, the music reached a crescendo, and there they were. Yes, there they were, the highlights of the show, the high point of the evening, the focal points of our lives.

Each of them held a large candle burning and lighting his way up on stage. They held the candles steadily and moved with exceptional grace and poise. I recognized them all. Not from this evening's performances. They had not performed. Not from some other public appearances. They had not appeared. I recognized them from my daily life. I knew them through part of my life.

They were the special children, the highlights, nay, the impetus of the evening—the HASC children. There was no applause. But there were tears, lots and lots of tears. Not sad tears. This was a very happy evening. Thousands had shown up; it was a success in every way. We were not sad about these children. On the contrary, we were awfully proud. They were tears of joy. Just looking at them, standing there with incredible reserve and dignity, did us all very, very proud.

Leibish was there, who else? He had been hand-picked by the HASC staff among just a few select participants in this last and most important feature of the concert. They knew what they were doing. One just had to glimpse him standing there, and one could not help but respect him. There was no fidgeting, no silly smirks, no self-consciousness, as I have seen on quite 'normal' people, who find themselves suddenly on stage, being watched by so many pairs of eyes.

As the performers came on stage, one by one, group by group, I saw them through a haze of happy tears. They danced and mingled with Leibish and his friends. They sang about a candle burning in the night, dispelling the darkness. And I sang about a child who has forever taken a special place in my heart, in my soul, in my life.

Epilogue

▼

My diary is going places! I find myself pondering the creation of this book. A little girl of eleven years of age starting a diary on a whim. Twenty-seven years ago a teacher took a moment to compliment a student on her writing abilities. She had taken the positive attitude and had overlooked the negative. She had ignored the misspellings (I hope I did not misspell this word) and forgotten that the student had spoken out of turn. Instead, she had taken notice of her strengths. Thank you, Mrs. Berenfeld, wherever you are!

Without Leibish there would be no book. My diary would have been very boring. I bet it would have been forgotten long ago, perhaps by the second or third entry. It would have been disposed of along with my other "great works" which I have undertaken over the years and long since forgotten.

Yes, Leibish has been my inspiration and not only with this book. In every facet of my life there is a little of Leibish, reminding me to smile at the girl with the unsightly harelip, at the crippled man in the wheelchair and, most importantly, to smile to myself and remember. Yes, Leibish, you are a special brother!

In the *Aron Kodesh* of my parents' *shul* stands a *Sefer Torah*, which outshines all the others. Newer, more extravagant ones have been added, but none could even come close to the *Sefer Torah* which my parents, with tender loving care and with most of their savings, have offered up to the One Above. As you look a little closer, and as your eyes become accustomed to the dim light, you will discern this little inscription on the velvet *mantele*.

Kisvu lachem es hashirah hazos. Hasefer hazeh nichtav al yedei Reb Chaim Weinfeld v'zugaso Moras Sarah l'zchus ul'mitzvah l'bnam hayakar Aryeh. Yehi ratzon shezchus haTorah taamod lo lo'ad, amen.

This *Sefer Torah*, according to the *mitzvah* of "*Kisvu lachem es hashirah hazos*," has been written through Reb Chaim Weinfeld and his wife Sara for the merit of their dear son Aryeh (Leibish). Let us pray that the merit of the Torah will stand by him forever.
Amen.

GLOSSARY

afikomen: part of the Passover Seder

Al Hanisim: *Chanukah* prayer

aleph-bais: Hebrew alphabet

aliyah: going up to read from the Torah

baal tefillah: cantor

baalas chessed: kind person

baalei simchah: hosts

bachur: teenage boy

badchan: jester at wedding

bais midrash: study hall

balabusta: homemaker

Baruch Hashem: Thank G-d

bashert: fated

benching: grace after meals

beracha: blessing

bikur cholim: visiting the sick

bimah: raised platform

Birchas Hatorah: blessing for the Torah

bitachon: faith

blech: aluminum covering for stove

bli ayin hora: free from evil eye

Borei Me'orei Ha'eish: blessing over the *Havdalah* candle

bris: circumcision

chachmos: cute stories

challos: Sabbath loaves

chametz: leavened bread

chas veshalom: Heaven forbid

chasan: bridegroom

chassan bachur: boy of marriageable age

chassidishe: *Chassidic*

chavrusa: study partner

cheder: elementary Torah school

chessed: kind act

Chol Hamoed: intermediary days of a holiday

cholent: Sabbath dish

Chumash: Five Books of Moses

chupah: wedding canopy

daven: pray

derhoiben: exalted

die alte heim: Homeland

dobosh-torto: Hungarian cream cake

dvar Torah: Torah thought

erev Pesach: Passover Eve

farbrengen: gathering

farshlafen: sleepy

frum: observant

Gan Eden: Paradise

257

gartel: traditional sash
gedolei hador: greatest Torah giants
gedolim: Torah giants
gelilah: wrapping the Torah scroll
Gemara: part of the Talmud
gilgul: reincarnation
goyishe: gentile
grammen: rhymes
gut Shabbos: Sabbath greeting
gut voch: post-Sabbath greeting
halachos: Jewish laws
Hallel: Holiday prayer
Hamalach Hagoel: bedtime prayer
Havdalah: ceremony marking the conclusion of Sabbath
heimish: of similar back ground
heisse chassid: devout *chassid*
Kaddish Yasom: Orphan's Prayer
kaddishel: son
kallah moid: a girl of marriageable age
kallah: bride
kashrus: kosher
kibbudim: honors
kichels: crackers
kiddush: blessing over wine; small celebration

kinderlach: children
Koheles: Ecclesiastes
kokosh: Hungarian-style coffe cake
Krias Hatorah: reading of the Torah
kugel: pudding
Lag b'Omer: Jewish Holiday
lashon hora: evil talk
Lashon Kodesh: ancient Hebrew; the holy tongue
lebedik, lebedikeit: lively, liveliness
lecht tzinden: candle lighting
Leshoni: Hebrew language workbook
Litvak: of Lithuanian origin
lo aleinu: Heaven forbid
Maariv: evening prayers
maasim tovim: good deeds
malach: angel
mashgiach: supervisor
matzoh: unleavened bread
mazel: luck
mechalel Shabbos: one who desecrates the Sabbath
mechutzaf: impudent one
mensch: man
menschele: little man
mesader kiddushin: rabbi officiating at wedding
meshuga: crazy
mezinikel: baby of the family

mezuman: quorum of three

Minchah: afternoon prayers

minhag: custom

minyan: a quorum of ten men

Mishlei: Proverbs

mishloach manos: food packages exchanged among friends on Purim

Mishnayos: part of the Talmud

mitzvos: good deeds

mohel: one who performs circumcision

Moshe Rabbeinu: Moses

Motzai Shabbos: Saturday night

nachas: joy

nebechs: unfortunates

neshamah: soul

niggun: tune

nosh: sweets

oilem: audience

oleh: one who reads from the Torah

parshah: portion of the Torah

passuk: Torah verse

peyos: earlocks

pekelech: baggies filled with goodies

Pesach: Passover

Pirkei Avos: Talmud tractate (dealing with ethics)

pshetl: traditional address by *bar-mitzvah* boy

Purim: Jewish Holiday

rav: rabbi

rebbe: Torah teacher

rebbetzin: rabbi's wife

redding shidduchim: matchmaking

Rosh Chodesh: start of lunar month

Seder: Passover ceremony

sefer: book

seudah: meal

Shabbaton: Sabbath spent with a group away from home

Shabbos tisch: Sabbath table

Shabbos: Sabbath

Shacharis: morning prayers

shadchanim: matchmakers

shaitel: wig

shalom zachar: Friday night ceremony for newborn son

shamesh: sexton in a synagogue

Shavuos: Jewish Holiday

Shema: prayer

Shemoneh Esrei: prayer

sheva brachos: seven days of festivities following a wedding

shidduch: match

Shir Hashirim: Song of Songs

shitah: custom

shiurim: lectures

259

Shomer Pesayim Hashem:
G-d guards the fools

shtetl: small East European town

shtreimel: fur hat usually worn by *chassidim*

shul: synagogue

Shulchan Aruch: Code of Jewish Law

siddur: prayer book

simchah: celebration

Simchas Torah: Jewish Holiday

sukkah: tabernacle

talmid chacham: Torah scholar

Tehillim: Psalms

tefillin: phylacteries

tichel: kerchief

Tisha b'Av: Ninth day in Av, a fast day

treifos: non-kosher food

trop: cantillation marks

tzedakah: charity

tzitzis: traditional fringed garments

tzu gutt und tzu leit: spiritual, yet worldly

tzugekimene: in-laws

upsherin: ceremonial cutting of hair

vachnacht: night before circumcision

veibele: young married woman

venohapochu: turned upside down

Yahadus: Judaism

Yamim Tovim: Jewish festivals

yeshivah: Jewish school

yetzer hora: evil inclination

yichud: being alone together

yichus: ancestry

Yiddishkeit: Judaism

yingele: little boy

Yom Tov: holiday

zatzal: of blessed memory

zchus: merit

zemiros: Sabbath melodies